Electrophysiological Correlates of Psychopathology

Advances in Biological Psychiatry

Vol. 9

Series Editors
J. Mendlewicz, Brussels, and *H. M. van Praag,* Bronx, N.Y.

S. Karger · Basel · München · Paris · London · New York · Sydney

3rd International Symposium on Clinical Neurophysiological Aspects of Psychopathological Conditions, Stockholm, June 28, 1981

Electrophysiological Correlates of Psychopathology

Volume Editors
C. Perris, Umeå; *D. Kemali,* Naples; *P. Flor-Henry,* Edmonton, Alta; *L. Vacca,* Naples

11 figures and 20 tables, 1982

S. Karger · Basel · München · Paris · London · New York · Sydney

Advances in Biological Psychiatry

National Library of Medicine, Cataloging in Publication
International Symposium on Clinical Neurophysiological Aspects of Psychopathological Conditions (3rd: 1981: Stockholm, Sweden)
Electrophysiological correlates of psychopathology / 3rd International Symposium on Clinical Neurophysiological Aspects of Psychopathological Conditions, Stockholm, June 28, 1981
Volume editors, C. Perris ... [et al.]. – Basel; New York: Karger, 1982.
(Advances in biological psychiatry; v. 9)
1. Electroencephalography – congresses 2. Evoked Potentials – congresses 3. Mental Disorders – diagnosis – congresses. I. Perris, Carlo II. Title III. Series
W1 AD44 v. 9 [WL 150 I615 1981e]
ISBN 3-8055-3525-2

Drug Dosage

The authors and the publisher have exerted every effort to ensure that drug selection and dosage set forth in this text are in accord with current recommendations and practice at the time of publication. However, in view of ongoing research, changes in government regulations, and the constant flow of information relating to drug therapy and drug reactions, the reader is urged to check the package insert for each drug for any change in indications and dosage and for added warnings and precautions. This is particularly important when the recommended agent is a new and/or infrequently employed drug.

Printed in Switzerland by Emmentaler Druck AG, Langnau
ISBN 3-8055-3525-2

Contents

CEEG/EP and Effects of Psychotropic Drugs

Acknowledgement

The publication of these proceedings has been sponsored by Lepetit SpA Milan

Foreword

The Third Symposium on Clinical Neurophysiological Aspects of Psychopathological Conditions was held at the same time as the Third World Congress of Biological Psychiatry in Stockholm, Sweden, in July 1981. This coincidence of timing was not accidental, but was planned as the aims our annual symposium and the general concepts of the Biological Psychiatry Congress are in accordance. In fact, these general concepts involve the analysis and interpretation of those biological factors which are at the basis of behaviour.

To study the interaction between subjectivity and behaviour, Biological Psychiatry does not exclude from its field the influence that the environment exercises over the emergence of observed phenomena. In order to interpret the pathogenesis of some manifestations of behaviour correctly, the biological approach not only selects and indicates phenomena which can be correlated but it also, from time to time, proposes various rules and strategies which can assist us to arrive at the desired results. That is, Biological Psychiatry must follow adaptable methods which are correctly applicable to systems with different degrees of complexity.

It is exactly at this point in the realm of these conceptual considerations that the annual meetings of our group take place. The previous two symposia – at Umeå and Capri – were held on the basis of the unanimous agreement on the part of the participants to delimit the object of research and the modalities for the organization and use of the analysis of the results. This principle is followed 'not as a step directly towards what we wish to know but more as a consolidating basis to allow us to start from what we know today'. This understanding has, in practice, given rise not only to an agreement on reciprocal work but has also suggested shared criteria that we can adopt both in our methods and evaluations. From these, as we shall see in the various papers of this symposium, an agreement on interests for future research has been devised.

The neurophysiological research applied to psychiatric problems implies a dangerous reductionism. The research into the possible correlation between software (psychopathological symptoms) and hardware (functional arrangements of cerebral activity) cannot be interpreted as corresponding relationships between one term and another, an isomorphism, that is, between aspects with homogeneous structures. This approach, on the one hand, might show information on the characteristics of signals from one or more areas of the brain and also evidence of the topographic relationships between these signals and the organization of the whole system. On the other hand, the above-mentioned research might indicate the incidence, in a syndrome, of environmental factors on the pathogenesis and the social and cultural significance which we can attribute to certain symptoms. This clinical relevance might manifest itself through the evidence of correlations between the syndrome, symptoms and modality of the whole assembly of the electrocortical activity.

In this symposium the lack of time has unfortunately compelled us to reduce the length of individual papers. In spite of this, the different contributions presented here have shown a common desire to achieve a deeper understanding of the still unknown aspects of psychiatric research by a clearere insight into and interpretation of the information which we have today.

Dargut Kemali

Adv. biol. Psychiat., vol. 9, pp. 1–7 (Karger, Basel 1982)

Studies in EEG Power and Coherence (8–13 Hz) in Depression Mania and Schizophrenia Compared to Controls

P. Flor-Henry[a], *Z. J. Koles*[b], *D. M. Tucker*[c]

[a]Alberta Hospital Edmonton, Edmonton, Alta., Canada; [b]Department of Biomedical Engineering, University of Alberta, Edmonton, Alta., Canada; [c]Department of Psychology, University of North Dakota, Grand Forks, N. Dak., USA

Depressive psychotics (n = 26), manic patients (n = 24), and schizophrenics (n = 19) were studied and compared to healthy controls (n = 30). All patients were unmedicated, and all subjects were consistent dextrals on the *Annett* [1970] Handedness Inventory. The diagnostic criteria applied to consecutive inpatient admissions were those of *Feighner* et al. [1972] and of *Taylor and Abrams* [1978]. The technical details of the power spectral analysis have been previously described [*Flor-Henry and Koles,* 1980; *Koles and Flor-Henry,* 1981]. The data to be described relate to EEG characteristics at T3, T4 and P3, P4 with unipolar montage against Cz reference, assessed under resting conditions (eyes open and closed) and during verbal cognitive activation (Vocabulary subtest) and spatial activation (Block Design subtest), both tasks taken from the Wechsler Adult Intelligence Scale. The statistical evaluation was estimated by the Mann-Whitney U test at the $p < 0.05$ probalility level.

The normal controls were selected so that the sex ratio (male/female = 1) should be balanced. The patients were not matched for either sex or age. The average ages of the three psychotic groups were comparable: depression = 35.5, mania = 38.2, and schizophrenia = 34.2 years. The average age of the controls was younger: 26.0 years. Interestingly, in these consecutive admissions, satisfying research criteria, the trend whereby females predominate in the affective syndromes and males in the

Table I. Power and coherence (8–13 Hz); (depression (n = 26) vs. normals (n = 30)

Eyes open – coherence PR–TR ↑ / *Eyes closed* – coherence TR–PL ↓	
Verbal	*Spatial*
Average power ↑	coherence PR–PL ↑
parietal, right and left	PR–TR
temporal, right and left	PR–TL
Average log, R/L coherence ratio:	TR–PL
normals negative	PL–TL
depression positive	

PR = Pariet. Right; TR = Tempor. Right; PL = Pariet. Left; TL = Tempor. Left

Table II. Power and coherence (8–13 Hz); mania (n = 24) vs. normals (n = 30)

Eyes open	*eyes closed*
Power: ↓ parietal, right and left	power: ↓ parietal, right and left
temporal, right and left	temporal, right and left
Average log, R/L coherence ratio:	average log, R/L coherence ratio:
Positive in normals	positive in normals
Negative in mania	negative in mania
	coherence: PR–TR ↓
Verbal	*spatial*
Power: ↓ parietal, right and left	power: ↓ parietal, right and left
temporal, right and left	temporal, right and left
Coherence: PR–PL ↓	coherence: TR–TL ↓
TR–TL	

PR = Pariet. Right; TR = Tempor. Right; PL = Pariet. Left; TL = Tempor. Left

schizophrenic syndromes once again emerged: male/female sex ratio for depression = 0.80, for mania = 0.85, and for schizophrenia = 1.30.

The average EEG characteristics of depression, mania, and schizophrenia were systematically compared to the controls; then the three psychoses were in turn compared to each other: mania vs. depression,

Table III. Power and coherence (8–13 Hz); schizophrenia (n = 19) vs. normals (n = 30)

Eyes open	*eyes closed*
Power: ↓ PL, TL, TR	power: ↓ parietal, right and left; temporal, right and left
Coherence: PL–PR, PL–TR ↓	
Verbal	*spatial*
Power: ↓ parietal, right and left; temporal, right and left	power: ↓ PL, TR
Average log, R/L parietal power ratio: Normals negative; Schizophrenia positive	coherence: TL–PR, TL–TR ↓

PR = Pariet. Right; TR = Tempor. Right; PL = Pariet. Left; TL = Tempor. Left

Table IV. Power and coherence (8–13 Hz); mania (n = 26) vs. depression (n = 24)

Eyes open	*eyes closed*
Coherence: PR–TR ↓	coherence: PR–TR ↓; PL–TL ↑
Average log, R/L coherence ratio: Positive in depression; Negative in mania	Average log, R/L coherence ratio: positive in depression; negative in mania
Verbal	*spatial*
Coherence: PR–TR, TR–TL ↓	coherence: all ↓ except PR–PL
Average log, R/L coherence ratio: Positive in depression; Negative in mania	

PR = Pariet. Right; TR = Tempor. Right; PL = Pariet. Left; TL = Tempor. Left

schizophrenia vs. mania, and schizophrenia vs. depression. The significant differences found for these various comparisons – relating to power and coherence in the alpha frequency band – are shown in tables I–VI. (In all tables the direction of the arrow indicates the direction ot the significant difference, $p < 0.05$, of the first group with respect to the second.)

Table V. Power and coherence (8–13 Hz); schizophrenia (n = 19) vs. mania (n = 24)

Eyes open	*eyes closed*
Coherence: TL–PR ↓	Average log, R/L parietal power ratio ↑ negative in mania positive in schizophrenia average log, R/L coherence ratio: negative in mania positive in schizophrenia
Verbal	*spatial*
Average log, R/L coherence ratio: Negative in mania Positive in schizophrenia	not significant

PR = Pariet. Right; TR = Tempor. Right; PL = Pariet. Left; TL = Tempor. Left

Table VI. Power and coherence (8–13 Hz); schizophrenia (n = 19) vs. depression (n = 26)

Eyes open			*Eyes closed*		
Coherence:	PR–TR TL–TR TL–PR	↓	power:	PL TL	↓
			coherence:	TL–TR	↓
Verbal			*spatial*		
Coherence:	TL–TR	↓	coherence:	TL–PR PL–TR PL–TL TL–TR	↓

PR = Pariet. Right; TR = Tempor. Right; PL = Pariet. Left; TL = Tempor. Left

Discussion

Power

In the eyes open condition schizophrenia shows an asymmetric reduction in alpha power, compared to the controls, suggesting an abnormal left hemisphere activation in schizophrenia (left parietal, left temporal, and right temporal). The average log of the right/left parietal power ratios in the eyes closed situation is positive in schizophrenia and negative in mania – this suggesting a greater degree of relative left hemisphere activation in schizophrenia and of right hemisphere activation in mania when these two psychoses are compared with each other. The characteristic abnormal activation of the left hemisphere in schizophrenia emerges again in the comparison with depression where the schizophrenia group exhibits a significant reduction of left parietal and temporal power. The reduction in right parietal alpha power previously reported in depression and mania [*Flor-Henry and Koles,* 1980], although still present as a trend in this new series, is no longer significant for depression. Here, both mania and schizophrenia (eyes closed) have bilateral alpha power suppression compared to controls. *Matousek* et al. [1981], however, have confirmed this pattern of right parietal alpha power reduction in 63 patients with endogenous depression compared to 317 controls, finding an opposite asymmetry in schizophrenia. A related finding is described by *Kemali* et al. [1981] who noted in 22 depressed patients a significant reduction of alpha mean power relative activity in the parietal regions (right < left) which does not occur in schizophrenia (n = 67) or controls (n = 65). The analysis of the distribution of the EEG amplitudes over the right and left hemispheres of depressed patients (n = 29) and controls (n = 20) carried out by *von Knorring and Goldstein* [1981] further emphasizes the specific involvement of the right hemisphere in depression. In normals, the distribution of the EEG amplitudes is Gaussian and unimodal 70 % of the time for the right and 80 % of the time for the left hemisphere. This distribution is abnormal and polymodal over the right hemisphere in 72 % of cases of depression.

Coherence

In the cognitively neutral conditions the intrahemispheric coherence on the right is increased in depression, compared to normals, and the opposite is found in mania. A left parietal focus of cerebral alteration with interhemispheric components is suggested in schizophrenia, where interhemispheric coherences between left and right parietal and left parietal and right temporal regions are reduced. The intrahemispheric coherence on the right is significantly lower in mania than in depression – implying in the former a greater degree of right hemisphere disorganization. On the other hand the average log of the right/left intrahemispheric ratio is significantly greater (and positive) in schizophrenia than it is in mania (where this ratio is negative). Further, *Tucker* et al. [1981], by factor analysis of the coherence matrix, in a normal subject studied weekly for a 6-

month period demonstrated a left frontal localization of maximal coherence during verbal and a right parietal zone of maximal coherence during spatial tasks. In the prior study of coherence relationships in normal dextral subjects during rest and verbal/spatial cognitive activation [*Flor-Henry and Koles,* 1980], the cognitive activation was found to be associated with a bilateral reduction of intrahemispheric coherence, with, however, a significant relative increase in the intrahemispheric coherence of the cognitively engaged hemisphere. Thus, the opposite right/left intrahemispheric ratios observed in schizophrenia and mania suggest opposite patterns of activation in schizophrenia and mania. At the level of coherence schizophrenia shows greater disorganization of both right intrahemispheric relations and interhemispheric systems than depression. During verbal cognitive activation the average log of the right/left intrahemispheric coherence ratio is negative in normals and positive in depressive patients suggesting (vide supra) more right hemisphere processing during speech in depression – a finding congruous with our previous reports of partial shifts of cognitive laterality during psychosis [*Flor-Henry and Koles,* 1980]. It is of interest that this ratio, during verbal task, is significantly different in mania (negative) compared to depression (positive) and in schizophrenia (positive) compared to mania (negative). Thus, a certain degree of right hemisphere processing during speech is suggested in both depression and schizophrenia, left hemisphere coherence relationships being similar in mania and normals.

Conclusions

The alpha power characteristics observed in this new series of endogenous psychoses – depressive, manic, and schizophrenic – suggest that an abnormal activation of the left hemisphere is associated with schizophrenia and of the right hemisphere with mania. The right and left intrahemispheric and interhemispheric coherence relationships found in the comparisons of each psychosis against controls and in the interpsychoses comparisons suggest a perturbation of right hemisphere systems in depression, a more profound such disturbance in mania and left parietal and interhemispheric disorganization in schizophrenia. Further, partial shifts of cognitive laterality during verbal tasks occur which may indicate a degree of right hemisphere language processing in both depression and schizophrenia.

References

Annett, M.: A classification of hand preference by association analysis. Br. J. Psychol. *61:* 303–321 (1970).

Feighner, J.P.; Robins, E.; Guze, S.; Woodruff, R.A., Jr.; Winokur, G.; Munoz, R.: Diagnostic criteria for use in psychiatric research. Archs. gen. Psychiat. *26:* 57–63 (1972).

Flor-Henry, P.; Koles, Z.J.: EEG studies in depression, mania and normals. Evidence for partial shifts of laterality in the affective psychosis. Adv. biol. Psychiat., vol. 4, pp. 21–43 (Karger, Basel 1980).

Kemali, D.; Vacca, L.; Marciano, F.; Nolfe, G.; Iorio, G.: CEEG findings in schizophrenics, depressives, obsessives, heroin addicts and normals; in Perris, Kemali, Vacca, Electroneurophysiology and psychopathology. Adv. biol. Psychiat., vol. 6, pp. 17–28 (Karger, Basel 1981).

Knorring, L. von; Goldstein, L.: Quantitative hemispheric EEG differences between healthy volunteers and depressed patients; in Analisi automatica dell'EEG nello studio della lateralizzazione cerebrale, Pisa 1981.

Koles, Z.J.; Flor-Henry, P.: Mental activity and the EEG: task and workload related effects. Med. biol. Eng. Comp. *19:* 185–194 (1981).

Matousek, M.; Capone, C.; Okawa, M.: Measurement of the interhemispherical differences as a diagnostic tool in psychiatry; in Perris, Kemali, Vacca, Electroneurophysiology and psychopathology. Adv. biol. Psychiat., vol. 6, pp. 76–80 (Karger, Basel 1981).

Taylor, M.A.; Abrams, R.: The prevalence of schizophrenia: a reassessment using modern diagnostic criteria. Am. J. Psychiat. *135:* 8 945–948 (1978).

Tucker, D.M.; Roth, D.L.; Sawler, B.G.: Factoring the intercoherence matrix: multivariate analysis of topographic coherence in the EEG. Ann. Meet. Int. Neuropsychol. Soc., Atlanta (in preparation).

P. Flor-Henry, MD, Alberta Hospital Edmonton, Box 307, Edmonton, Alta. (Canada)

Adv. biol. Psychiat., vol. 9, pp. 8–12 (Karger, Basel 1982)

Automatic EEG Analysis in the Diagnosis and Treatment of Organic Psychosyndrome Due to Brain Atrophy and Normotensive Hydrocephalus

M. Matousek, C. Blomstrand, C. Wikkelsø

Departments of Clinical Neurophysiology and Neurology, Sahlgren University Hospital, Gothenburg, Sweden

Introduction

According to previous observations, introduction of a shunt into the ventricular system has a good therapeutic effect not only in hypertensive but also in normotensive hydrocephalus. A substantial improvement of the organic psychosyndrome can be achieved in about 50 % of the patients [*Katzman,* 1977] but the therapeutic effect is minimal in other patients. In view of the risk of complications [*Greenberg* et al., 1977], the need for reliable prognostic criteria is obvious. In this study, a combination of various diagnostic procedures in connection with a cerebrospinal fluid tap-test [*Wikkelsø* et al., 1982] was employed in order to establish more accurate indications for the neurosurgical treatment. Thus, the study gave a unique opportunity to compare EEG findings with results of other examinations, applied simultaneously, in a well-defined material. The results based on automatic EEG analysis are presented in this paper.

Patients and Methods

Altogether 27 patients with normotensive hydrocephalus (n = 15) or cerebral atrophy and dementia of different origin (n = 12), aged from 37 to 76 years, were repeatedly examined. Among the patients with hydrocephalus, a vascular of traumatic origin was suspected in 53 % of cases, the cause being unknown in the remaining cases. Axial tomography showed an enlarged ventricular system in all patients (Ewans index 0.37, SD 0.05). The pressure of the cerebrospinal fluid was normal (mean 13.43 cm H_2O, SD 5.9). The patients were also examined by lumbar isotope cisternography and routine cerebrospinal fluid an blood examinations to exclude inflammatory diseases and metabolic disorders. The clinical symptoms such as impairment of intellectual functions, slow thinking, memory disturbances, passivity, sleepiness and urinary incontinence were registered on a three-point scale, and the total score was used to evaluate the clinical state. Four psychometric tests (Raven, Bingley's memory test, Identical Forms Test and reaction time measurement) were also applied.

A cerebrospinal tap-test was performed in all patients. The patients were examined at the same hour during 2 consecutive days, before and after withdrawal of 40–50 ml of cerebrospinal fluid by lumbar puncture. A temporary improvement, considered as a positive prognostic sign [*Wikkelsø* et al., 1982], was noted in 11 of the hydrocephalus patients.

The patients with normotensive hydrocephalus were referred to ventriculoperitoneal shunt operation, the indication being based on the following criteria: (1) typical clinical picture with progressive mental deterioration, gait disturbance and urinary incontinence; (2) characteristic finding at axial tomography with diminished periventricular attenuation, dilated temporal horns and no signs of cortical atrophy, and (3) retention of isotope in the lateral ventricles for 24 h or more, together with a block of flow over the cerebral hemispheres at isotope cisternography. To register the therapeutic effect, all the examinations were repeated 3 months after the neurosurgery.

Altogether 62 EEGs, taken in both treated and untreated patients, were analyzed in derivations F7-T3, F8-T4, T3-T5, T4-T6, P3-O1 and P4-O2. Photic stimulation was used in the beginning of each examination to standardize the vigilance level. The patient was then left undisturbed, lying down with his eyes closed, for 5 min. The amplitude of the activity in various bands was calculated in 12 selected epochs of 5 s duration. The epochs with artefacts and sleep activity were automatically rejected using a procedure developed by *Arvidsson* et al. [1977]. The degree of abnormality was assessed visually and also by 'normality quotients', comparing the spectra with those found in the normal population [*Matousek and Petersén,* 1973]. A continuous recording of 5 min duration was used to measure the vigilance level. The coefficients derived by means of multiple regression in a training material with well-defined alert and sleep activity were employed [*Matousek and Petersén,* 1979]. The measurement was done separately for each 5 s epoch, and the mean, variance and trend was calculated for the whole 5-min period.

Results

Examination before Treatment

Significant correlation between the amplitude of the EEG activity and the total clinical score was found in all frequency bands except slow α-activity (7.5–9.5 Hz). More pronounced clinical symptoms were associated with increase of activity below 7.5 Hz ($p<0.05$) and with decrease of activities above 9.5 Hz ($p<0.05$ for α_2 and β_1, $p<0.01$ for β_2). The findings were almost identical in all EEG derivations used.

To obtain information on the relevance of different methods of examination, the indicator with the highest correlation to the total clinical score was chosen to represent each method. As shown in figure 1, both EEG indicators (normality ratio and mean vigilance level) were closely

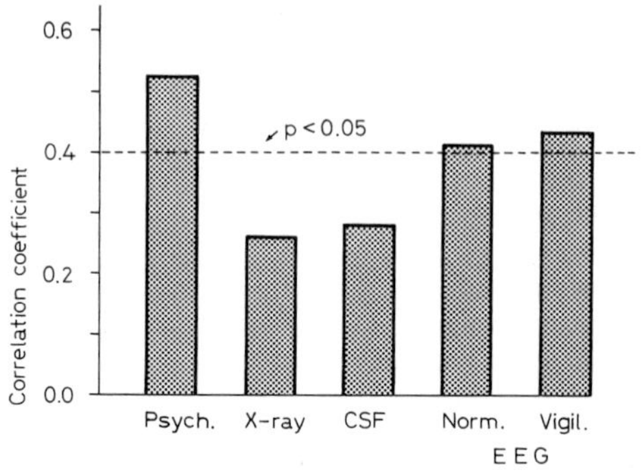

Fig. 1. Correlation between the results of different examination procedures and the total clinical score (n = 27). The indicator with the highest correlation was chosen to represent each method: Bingley's memory test, Ewans index, cerebrospinal fluid pressure, EEG normality ratio and mean vigilance level (see Methods).

related to the psychic state while the size of the ventricles (Ewans index) and cerebrospinal fluid pressure were not significantly correlated to the clinical score.

Changes after Treatment

The outcome of the treatment was defined as the difference between the total scores at the first and last examination. Of 15 treated patients, 8 of them displayed a clear improvement according to the clinical score. As shown in figure 2, diminished Ewans index as well as decrease of the cerebrospinal fluid pressure was noted after neurosurgery in all cases. However, there were no significant differences between the improved and nonimproved patients. In contrast to this, both EEG indicators were correlated to the clinical outcome of the treatment. In particular, the 'normality ratio' increased or decreased parallel with clinical improvement or deterioration. The vigilance level decreased in the paients in whom the treatment was not successful. The differences are statistically significant in both cases (Wilcoxon test, $p < 0.05$).

Prediction of the Therapeutic Outcome

The outcome of the treatment was correlated to the results before and after the test (see Methods). The changes of the 'normality ratio' after the test displayed a significant correlation to the outcome of therapy (Wilcoxon test, $p < 0.05$).

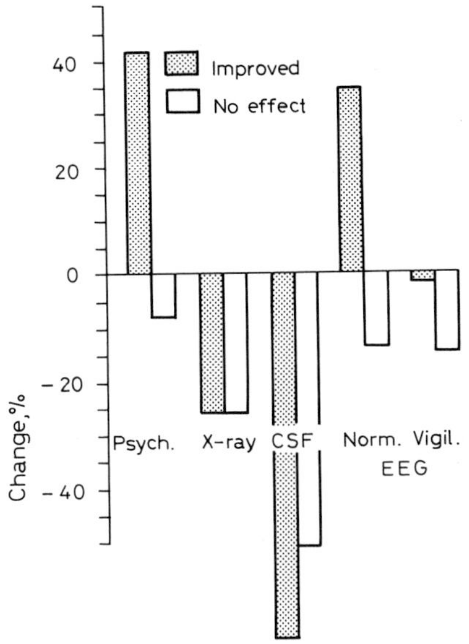

Fig. 2. The outcome of neurosurgical treatment as reflected by different examination procedure (the same indicators as in figure 1). In contrast to Ewans index and cerebrospinal fluid pressure, both EEG measures reflect the differences between the improved (n = 8) and nonimproved (n = 7) patients ($p < 0.05$, Wilcoxon test).

Discussion and Conclusion

The study of patients with an organic psychosyndrome shows that the method, which is based on EEG spectra, is advantageous as an aid to assess the clinical state, the prognosis, and the effect of treatment. In particular, the previously described 'normality quotients' [*Matousek and Petersén,* 1973] seem to be useful in connection with the cerebrospinal fuid tap-test. The results of the study suggest that EEG together with clinical observation and certain psychological tests [published separately: *Wikkelsø* et al., 1982] can be employed to establish relevant selection criteria for neurosurgical treatment when a more extensive material becomes available.

The observations after the treatment illustrated well that the magnitude of the organic lesion is not directly related to the intensity of clinical symptoms. The improvement of the gross pathology was not always followed by clinical improvement. The results of the EEG vigilance surements are of interest in this context. The findings suggest that the shifts of vigilance, and not exclusively the organic changes as such, may be responsible for some of the clinical symptoms connected with organic brain lesions.

References

Arvidsson, A.; Friberg, S.; Matousek, M.; Petersén, I.: Automatic selection of data for quantitative EEG analysis. Electroenceph. clin. Neurophysiol. *43:* 43 (1977).

Greenberg, J.O.; Shenkin, H.A.; Adam, R.: Idiopathic normal pressure hydrocephalus – a report of 73 patients. J. Neurol. Neurosurg. Psychiat. *40:* 336–341 (1977).

Katzman, R.: Normal pressure hydrocephalus; in Wells, Dementia (Davis, Philadelphia 1977).

Matousek, M.; Petersén, I.: Automatic evaluation of EEG background activity by means of age-dependent EEG quotients. Electroenceph. clin. Neurophysiol. *35:* 603–612 (1973).

Matousek, M.; Petersén, I.: Automatic measurement of the vigilance level and its possible application in psychopharmacology. Pharmakopsychiatr. Neuro-Psychopharmakol.. *12:* 148–154 (1979).

Wikkelsø, C.; Andersson, H.; Blomstrand, C.; Lindquist, G.: The clinical effect of lumbar puncture in normal pressure hydrocephalus (in press, 1982).

M. Matousek, MD, Department of Clinical Neurophysiology,
Sahlgren Hospital, S-41345 Gothenburg (Sweden)

Adv. biol. Psychiat., vol. 9, pp. 13–19 (Karger, Basel 1982)

Clinical and Quantitative Electroencephalographic and Symptomatological Differences between Italian and Swedish Depressives[1]

C. Perris[a], *K. Monakhov*[b], *S. Nikiforov*[b], *D. Kemali*[c], *L. Vacca*[c]

[a] University of Umeå, Department of Psychiatry, Umeå, Sweden; [b] Academy of Medical Science, Institute of Psychiatry, Laboratory of Neurophysiology, Moscow, USSR; [c] University of Naples, First Medical School, Institute of Psychiatry, Naples, Italy

Introduction

Clinical and quantitative electroencephalographic (CEEG) data have been obtained from a group of Swedish and Italian depressed patients within the frame of a long-term international collaborative study, which is still ongoing [*Perris* et al., 1978, 1981; *Monakhov* et al., 1979]. The present article deals with some preliminary results of this investigation.

Evidence supporting the hypothesis that statistically significant relationships may occur between depressive symptoms and EEG characteristics as well as between interhemispheric organization and depression has been reported in the literature [*d'Elia and Perris,* 1973; *Goldstein,* 1975; *Flor-Henry* et al., 1979; *Perris,* 1975; *Perris* et al., 1978; *Monakhov* et al., 1979; *Perris and Monakhov,* 1979; *Monakhov and Perris,* 1980]. It has, also been shown that the EEG of depressed patients differs from that of healthy controls [*Flor-Henry* et al., 1979; *Kemali* et al., 1981].

In a recent cross-cultural study between matched groups of Swedish and Italian depressed patients, similar also for the severity of the illness according to both the WHO/s ICD-8 and the 'Multi-Aspects Classification Model' (MACM) [*Ottosson and Perris,* 1973], some symptomatological differences between the two groups have been detected. They have been interpreted as being very likely due to cultural determinants.

[1] Supported in part by funds of the Italian National Council of Research CT 8100086.04 and the Swedish Medical Research Council (grants no 21X-5244 and 21X-2568).

Since it has been shown [*Perris* et al., 1978; *Perris and Monakhov,* 1979; *Monakhov and Perris,* 1980] that significant correlations occur between symptomatological and EEG measures, it can be expected that patients with a similar clinical diagnosis but different in symptomatology, differ also in EEG characteristics. This study was carried out to find a preliminary answer to this question.

Patients and Methods

37 Swedish and 37 Italian depressed in-patients matched for sex, and age and similar in clinical diagnosis both according to the ICD-8 and the MACM [*Ottosson and Perris,* 1973] have participated in the study. They had been previously included in a study of possible transcultural symptomatological differences [*Perris* et al., 1981] where details about their collection are reported. The composition of the series in shown in table I.

Resting EEG records were obtained in similar standardized conditions in Umeå and Naples. Six monopolar leads registered from symmetrical frontal, central and occipital areas according to the 10–20 system (F_2, F_3, C_4, C_3, O_2, O_1), have been used.

The analysis of the records was carried out at the Department of Neurophysiology in Moscow by means of a computer Mitra 15, using the basic principles of the systemic structural analysis of the EEG as reported elsewhere [*Perris* et al., 1978]. 60 s of artefact-free records have been used for the computer analysis.

The programme consists of three main steps: first the selection of primary EEG characteristics. In this case the following three EEG primary characteristics: the mean wave amplitude (μV), the mean wave period (ms) and the mean values of the index (duration of fragments of frequencies laying in each band calculated in precentage of the total EEG epoch of 60 s have been extracted for each of the six leads explored and for each of the conventional EEG frequency bands: alpha, beta, theta. All these values (total amount $n = 54$ characteristics for each EEG) have also been normalized. The second step includes a multifactorial analysis (modified eigen-vector technique) to describe and compress all the EEG variables mentioned above. The third part of the programme comprises a modified discriminant function analysis to investigate the distribution of the factors according to the concept of 'the neurofunctional system' [*Perris* et al., 1978; *Monakhov* et al., 1979], wich may differentiate two groups of patients in an experiment. Following the MACM criteria, used both in Umeå and Naples the patient's present status was classified into 'psychotic' and 'nonpsychotic' (table I).

The Zung's Self-Rating Scale for Depression (SDS) [*Zung,* 1965] and a subscale [*Perris* et al., 1981] of the Comprehensive Psychopathological Rating Scale (CPRS) [*Åsberg* et al., 1978] were also used for rating single depressive symptoms.

Results and Comments

The normalized mean values of primary EEG variables of Swedish and Italian depressed patients are shown in table II. The final EEG results from

Table I. The series

Patients	n	Sex M/F	Age, years $\bar{x} \pm$ S.D.	WHO 296/300.4	Psychotic/ nonpsychotic
Swedish	37 (36)	15/22	41 ± 10.2	20/17	13/24
Italian	37 (32)	15/22	41 ± 10.7	19/18	10/27
					n.s.

The number of EEGs suitable for EEG analysis are shown in parentheses.

Table II. Mean values of primary EEG characteristics of Italian (n = 37) and Swedish (n = 37) patients

Leads	Index			Period			Amplitude		
	beta	alpha	theta	beta	alpha	theta	beta	alpha	theta
O_l									
Italian	23.9	64.9	9.9	57.0	99.8	161.4	10.7	19.4	20.5
Swedish	34.6*	54.4*	6.8	53.9*	99.2**	159.1**	14.8*	26.8*	29.3*
O_r									
Italian	25.4	64.3	9.1	56.4	99.2	161.3	11.0	20.0	20.6
Swedish	35.5*	56.5	5.6	54.1*	99.0	156.4**	15.2**	28.5*	30.8*
C_l									
Italian	24.1	60.8	13.5	55.8	101.0	162.0	9.0	16.2	18.2
Swedish	39.9*	49.2*	8.4	53.2**	99.5**	156.4**	14.7**	24.8*	29.9*
C_r									
Italian	25.0	59.8	14.0	56.0	101.3	162.1	9.0	16.4	18.3
Swedish	44.6*	45.6*	6.6*	52.6*	97.8*	157.3	14.7*	25.3*	29.3*
F_l									
Italian	28.2	58.6	11.6	54.7	101.1	159.8	9.2	16.2	19.0
Swedish	45.2*	44.2*	6.4*	52.0*	98.0*	156.0	12.3*	20.6	26.1*
F_r									
Italian	27.6	59.2	11.5	54.6	101.1	162.0	9.9	17.5	21.6
Swedish	45.4*	43.6*	7.0*	52.0*	98.1*	157.5	12.2*	20.2**	25.7**

Index = Each band percentage over 60 s; Amplitude = mean amplitude (μV); Period = mean wave duration (ms).
* Significant ($p < 0.01$); ** not significant ($p > 0.05$); the rest uncertainity ($0.01 < p < 0.05$).

Table III. EEG data from discriminant analysis in Swedish and Italian depressives

EEG parameters	Weight of vectors, δ					
	I	II	III	IV	V	VI
Index, %	−0.11	+0.09	*+1.11*	*−0.58*		
Amplitude, μV	+0.2	−0.05	−0.09	−0.32		
Period, ms	+0.2	−0.28	−0.16	*+0.75*	+0.19	*+0.34*

General vectors are indicated; basic values are normalized.
δ = Standard deviation.
All values are statistically significant.
Figures in italics indicate highest values of significance.

Table IV. Symptomatological differences between Swedish and Italian depressives (mean values ± SD)

	Swedish (n = 37)		Italian (n = 37)	P
CPRS-depression subscale				
Inability to feel	1.8 ± 0.8	>	1.1 ± 0.8	<0.0004
Hypochondriasis	0.3 ± 0.6	<	1.0 ± 0.9	<0.0006
Reduced appetite	1.0 ± 0.8	<	1.0 ± 0.9	<0.05
Reduced speech	1.3 ± 1.0	<	1.6 ± 0.9	<0.0001
Slowness of movement	0.8 ± 0.8	<	1.4 ± 0.7	<0.0007
Agitation	0.5 ± 0.8	>	0.2 ± 0.6	<0.006
Zung SDS				
Tachycardia	2.2 ± 1.0	>	1.7 ± 0.8	<0.03
Agitation	2.8 ± 0.9	>	2.0 ± 1.1	<0.001

the discriminant function analysis of the general factors describing the primary EEG characteristics (index, amplitude, period) in the two groups of patients are presented in table III. The weights of the vectors, which describe the three elementary EEG variables selected in the present study, are expressed as values of the standard deviation (sigma). It can be seen that, with respect to the Mahalanobis coefficient (distance between the two groups at the discriminant analysis) in the two groups, there are differences in all vectors (they also indicate the tendency of EEG characteristics to increase or decrease in each experimental group) and that the third, fourth and sixth vectors show the highest values. This last finding suggests that the

Table V. Clinical and EEG main differences between Italian and Swedish depressed patients

Symptoms	Rating scales	Vectors	EEG parameters and leads		EEG symptom differences, Italian/Swedish
Inability to feel	CPRS		index	$\uparrow\delta C_R$ $\downarrow\beta C_R$ $\downarrow\delta C_L$ $\uparrow\beta C_L$	
Agitation	CPRS	IV			<
Tachycardia	SDS		amplitude	$\uparrow\beta F_L$ $\uparrow\alpha C_L$ $\uparrow\delta C_L$	
Agitation	SDS			$\downarrow\beta O_L$ $\downarrow\alpha O_L$ $\downarrow\delta O_R$	
Hypochondriasis	CPRS				
Reduced appetite	CPRS	III	index	$\downarrow\beta F_{LR}$ $\uparrow\alpha F_{LR}$ $\uparrow\beta O_{LR}$ $\downarrow\alpha O_{LR}$	
Reduced speech	CPRS	IV	period	$\uparrow\delta F_{LR}$ $\downarrow\delta O_{LR}$	>
Slowness movement	CPRS	VI	period	$\uparrow\delta C_R$ $\uparrow\delta F_R$ $\downarrow\delta F_L$	

Only the differences with the highest degree of distance are indicated (Gen. Mahalanobis $D^2 = 121.5$). Greek letters = EEG conventional frequency band; C = central; F = frontal; O = occipital; CPRS = Comprehensive psychopathological Rating Scale [*Åsberg* et al., 1978]; SDS = Self-Rating Scale for Depression [*Zung*, 1965]. ↑ indicates tendency to increase and ↓ to decrease of the corresponding EEG characteristic.

last-mentioned vectors play a higher role in the discrimination between the two groups (table III). In table IV the symptomatological differences between Italian and Swedish patients as found in the previous study are presented [*Perris* et al., 1981].

In table V the symptoms with different scores between Italian and Swedish depressives and the highest significant EEG differences between the two groups are indicated, but the direct correlation between single symptoms and EEG characteristics is not shown. In table V the data are lined up in such a way that in the upper part the symptoms are shown in which Italian patients scored less than Swedish and also the EEG measures were lower. In the lower part are indicated the symptoms and EEG variables with higher values in the Italian group and also the EEG frequency band and leads in which the vectors show the highest difference and the largest discriminant function level. The high significance of these differences (D^2 coefficient = 121.5) is understandable taking into account that, with the method used and for the number of factors considered, the limit value of the coefficient of distance (the Mahalanobis Gen. D^2 coefficient) is 22.04. For each EEG elementary characteristic, the vectors indicate the tendency of the EEG measures to increase or decrease in the Italian and Swedish group.

To exemplify: in the upper part of table V, in the first line vector IV describes that in the Italian group the tendency of the theta index in the right central area to increase is much less than in the Swedish group, and that the distance between the two groups at the discriminant function is very high (D^2 coefficient 121.5). In synthesis, the findings, at the present time, indicate that the Italian depressives when compared with the Swedish ones show symptomatological and EEG differences.

The finding that there are EEG differences between the Swedish and the Italian patients, despite being alike in age, sex, clinical diagnosis and severity of illness, is in line with our expectations. In fact, it seems that EEG characteristics, for example, those taken into account in the present article, are possibly correlated with the symptomatology present at the moment of the EEG investigation and not with the basic clinical diagnosis [*Perris* et al., 1978; *Monakhov and Perris,* 1980]. The results of our study on that point confirm the needs of a careful analysis of the symptoms presented by the patients at the time of an EEG investigation if results obtained in different centers have to be compared or pooled together. In fact, our results show that demographic variables such age and sex, clinical characteristics such as a traditional diagnostic label, and an evaluation of the severity of the illness are not enough to make two different series completely comparable. As far as the EEG and symptoms correlations are concerned, they will be evaluated in further investigations in a larger group of patients coming from different sociocultural environments.

Summary

A quantitative analysis of the EEGs has been done in Swedish and Italian depressed patients, matched for sex, age, clinical diagnosis and severity of illness. The findings indicate that some EEG characteristics are different between the two groups. Moreover, Swedish and Italian depressed patients have also shown quantitative differences in some symptoms present at the moment of the EEG investigation. The data confirm our previous results and are also of interest for further investigation in order to verify some possible correlations between single symptoms of the depressive syndrome and EEG variables in groups of patients coming from different etnical and sociocultural environments.

References

Åsberg, M.; Perris, C.; Schalling, D.; Sedvall, G.: The CPRS: development and application of a Psychiatric Rating Scale. Acta psychiat. scand., suppl. 271 (1978).

D'Elia, G.; Perris, C.: Cerebral functional dominance and depression. Acta psychiat. scand. *49:* 191–197 (1973).

Flor-Henry, P.; Koles, Z.J.; Howarth, B.G.; Burton, L.: Neurophysiological studies of schizophrenia, mania and depression; in Gruzelier, Flor-Henry, Hemisphere asymmetries of function in psychopathology, pp. 189–222 (Elsevier, Amsterdam 1979).

Goldstein, L.: Interhemispheric EEG amplitude analysis in man under various behavioural status. Proc. 2nd Symp. Study Group EEG Methodology Jongny-Sur-Vey 1975, pp. 159–170.

Kemali, D.; Vacca, L.; Marciano, F.; Nolfe, G.; Iorio, G.: CEEG findings in schizophrenia, depressives, obsessives, heroin addicts and normals. Adv. biol. Psychiat. vol. 6, pp. 17–28 (1981).

Monakhov, K.; Perris, C.: Neurophysiological correlates of depressives symptomatology. Neuropsychobiology *6:* 269–279 (1980).

Monakhov, K.; Perris, C.; Botskarev, V.K.; Knorring, L. von; Nikiforov, A.: Functional interhemispheric differences in relation to various psychopathological components of depressive syndrome. A pilot international study. Neuropsychobiology *5:* 143–155 (1979).

Ottosson, J.O.; Perris, C.: Multidimensional classification of mental disorders. Psychobiol. Med. *3:* 238–243 (1973).

Perris, C.: EEG tecniques in the measurement of the severity of depressive syndromes. Neuropsychobiology *1:* 16–25 (1975).

Perris, C.; Eiseman, M.; Eriksson, V.; Perris, H.; Kemali, D.; Amati, A.; Del Vecchio, M.; Vacca, L.: Transcultural aspects of depressive symptomatology. Psychiatria clin. *14:* 69–80 (1981).

Perris, C.; Monakhov, K.: Depressive symptomatology and systemic. Structural analysis of the EEG, in Gruzelier, Flor-Henry, Hemisphere asymmetries of function in psychopathology, pp. 223–226 (Elsevier, North Holland 1979).

Perris, C.; Monakhov, K.; Knorring L. von; Botskarev, V.; Nikiforov, A.: Systemic structural analysis of the electroencephalogram of depressed patients. General principles and preliminary results of an international collaborative study. Neuropsychobiology *4:* 207–228 (1978).

Zung, W.K.: A self rating depression scale. Archs gen. Psychiat. *12:* 63–70 (1965).

C. Perris, MD, Department of Psychiatry, University of Umeå, S-90185 Umeå (Sweden)

Adv. biol. Psychiat., vol. 9, pp. 20–27 (Karger, Basel 1982)

Central Components of the Orienting Response (EEG Reactivity) in Acute and Former Schizophrenics, Neurotics, and Normals

Martha Koukkou, Marianne Bigler, D. Lehmann

Research Department, University Hospital of Psychiatry, Zurich, Switzerland

Introduction

Several years ago we started collecting data on EEG reactivity (i. e., on the central components of the orienting response) of different psychopathological conditions. Until now, we have presented results on acute schizophrenics, former schizophrenics, and normal controls [*Koukkou,* 1980a, b, 1982]. In this report we present results on a group of neurotics as compared to the three other groups.

These studies are based on two main observations: (1) in an information processing approach of the orienting response [*Öhman,* 1979], the characteristics (form, strength, and duration) of the EEG reactivity to stimuli indicate the result of the initial interpretation of the incoming information by the central nervous system [*Koukkou,* 1980b], and (2) the stimulus-induced EEG brain state after the initial interpretation is decisive for the following (cognitive) processing of the received information [*Lehmann,* 1980]. Therefore, the central components of the orienting response reflect a fundamental mechanism of the organism for its communication with the environment. In the previous publications we tested the hypothesis that the communication deficit during productive schizophrenic symptoms is reflected in a deviation of the EEG components of the orienting response (deviant EEG reactivity) and that this deviation is normalized during a good clinical remission. Our results confirmed this hypothesis. In the present report we examine the hypothesis that the cognitive deficit, which may be hypothesized to exist during neurotic symptomatology [*Gossop,* 1981], is reflected in a deviant EEG reactivity to stimuli, but that this deviation differs from that seen in acute and former schizophrenics.

In the previous reports we measured the EEG reactivity with the stimulus-induced changes of the centroid (distribution mean) values of frequency bands of the power spectra [*Lehmann and Koukkou,* 1974]. In this paper, in addition to centroids, we use integrated spectral band power as measure of the EEG reactivity in order to examine whether within the same frequency band different spectral EEG parameters separate different psychopathological groups.

Methods

The groups of acute schizophrenics, former schizophrenics, and normal controls have been described previously [*Koukkou,* 1980a, b]. We repeat that the group of *acute* schizophrenics consisted of new hospital admissions during a *first* acute manifestation of productive schizophrenic symptoms. The patients had, before recording, never received antipsychotic medication (n = 22, 14 males, 8 females, age 25.8 ± 5.7 years). The group of *former* schizophrenics consisted of persons who had been discharged from the hospital after a complete clinical remission of a first acute schizophrenic episode. The EEG recording was done 3 months after termination of all antipsychotic medication (n = 22, 14 males, 8 females, age 26.3 ± 4.2 years). The group of normal *controls* consisted of volunteers (n = 20, 14 males and 6 females, age 26.7 ± 3.8 years). The group of *neurotics* consisted of persons who had been hospitalized because of a neurotic breakdown, who had been discharged from the hospital after a reduction of the symptoms which had led to the hospitalization, and who had been free of drugs for more than 3 months at the time of the EEG examination. Thus, at the time of the EEG recording the group of neurotics showed similarities in their 'career' as psychiatric patients with the group of former schizophrenics. The 21 persons (13 males, 8 females, age 29.2 ± 4.7 years) included in this group had been hospitalized because of depressive symptoms (10 cases), anxiety (7 cases), phobic symptoms (2 cases), and obsessive-compulsive symptoms (2 cases).

The study was designed to produce several EEG epochs before and after the presentation of auditory information which the subjects were asked to attend [for details see *Koukkou,* 1980a, b]. Here we analyze data obtained (1) while resting with eyes closed, (2) after the instruction to close the previously opened eyes, and (3) after presentation of two short, meaningless sentences made up from regular words. The EEG of the following conditions (EEG epochs) will be presented: 80 s resting with closed eyes (= R), 20 s after the instruction to close the previously opened eyes (= 1), 20 s immediately after the presentation of the first sentence (= 2), 40 s after condition 2 (= 3), 20 s immediately after the presentation of the second sentence (= 4), and 40 s after condition 4 (= 5). For the two sentences we consider two different EEG time epochs after the presentation in order to examine the differences in the duration of the EEG reactivity between the four subject groups. All data were recorded on paper and FM tape and collected with eyes closed except during the instruction to open the eyes.

Table I. Mean values and standard deviations of centroids and integrated power of the 8- to 13-Hz frequency band, for the 6 conditions (see text)

	Centroid						Integrated power					
	R	1	2	3	4	5	R	1	2	3	4	5
Normal controls												
Mean	10.31	10.54	10.44	10.41	10.42	10.41	174.3	145.8	130.0	154.0	143.9	151.9
SD	0.38	0.33	0.26	0.28	0.31	0.33	116	81	91	108	91	100
n	20	20	19	19	20	20	20	19	19	20	20	20
Former schizophrenics												
Mean	10.28	10.49	10.42	10.43	10.41	10.40	134.4	132.1	120.4	130.7	131.1	133.2
SD	0.34	0.40	0.38	0.39	0.38	0.38	69	67	68	66	76	69
n	22	22	21	19	20	22	22	21	19	20	22	22
Neurotics												
Mean	10.21	10.34	10.34	10.30	10.30	10.30	147.7	125.9	114.8	128.1	113.7	123.3
SD	0.43	0.33	0.42	0.41	0.40	0.37	66	74	60	66	56	64
n	21	21	20	20	21	21	21	21	20	20	21	21
Acute schizophrenics												
Mean	10.31	10.34	10.42	10.36	10.32	10.32	138.5	143.6	116.4	129.7	114.7	120.4
SD	0.34	0.30	0.31	0.30	0.33	0.35	68	74	60	62	64	61
n	22	19	22	19	21	19	22	22	19	21	19	19
p	0.82	0.17	0.82	0.67	0.60	0.67	0.40	0.33	0.91	0.68	0.50	0.55
Eta^2	0	6	1	1	2	2	1	1	0	1	3	2

p and eta^2 values of the Anova.

After the exclusion of recordings with artefacts after investigation of the paper records, the EEG was off-line analog low-pass filtered at 26 Hz and A/D converted (256 s/s/channel). Using a hanning window, power spectra were computed with a resolution of 0.25 Hz, using a Fourier transformation based program by *Stassen*. Then, the data were computed for segments of 20 s omitting values below the 2-Hz band.

For the reduction of the resulting frequency spectral distributions into few descriptors, distribution means [centroids, *Lehmann and Koukkou,* 1974], and integrated power were computed for conventional frequency bands. The two parameters were computed for each subject and channel. In this report, because of space limits, data from the left parietooccipital lead (all subjects were self-reported dextrals) in the 8- to 13-Hz band will be presented. An analysis of variance was carried out on each parameter and each condition. Then, for each subject and parameter the EEG reactivity was computed, defined as the amount of change of

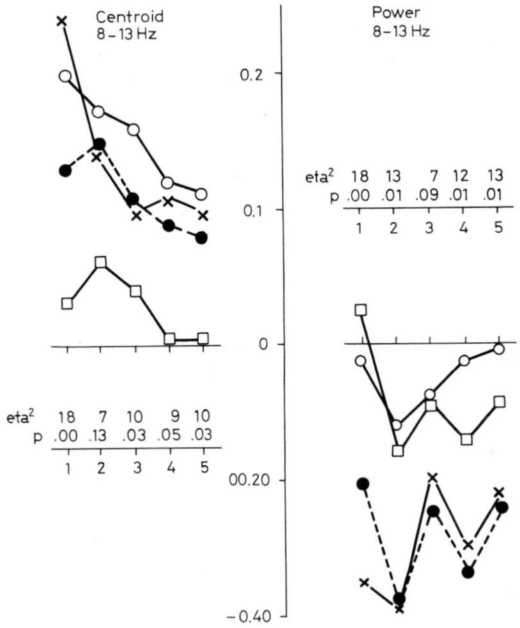

Fig. 1. Mean values of EEG reactivity (centroid and integrated power differences to baseline, vertical) in the 8- to 13-Hz frequency band, the four subject groups and the five conditions (horizontal). p and eta^2 values of Anova. For details see text. □ = acute schizophrenics; ○ = former schizophrenics; ● = neurotics; × = control subjects.

each parameter (centroid or integrated power) between the initial resting EEG epoch (R) and the EEG epoch of the five other conditions. Analysis of variance was carried out on each of the reactivity measures and on each of the conditions. The significance of the induced EEG change (EEG reactivity) within each group was tested with the paired Wilcoxon test.

Results

Centroids and Integrated Power during the Six Conditions

Table I gives the mean values and standard deviations of the centroids and the integrated power of the 8- to 13-Hz frequency band during resting and the five other conditions for the four subject groups. The results of the

Anova indicate that there are no significant differences, as measured with these parameters and this frequency band, between the four groups.

EEG Reactivity Measured with the Centroid

The analysis of variance (fig. 1) showed significant results for all EEG reactivities (p values between 0.05 and 0.001 and eta^2 values between 9 and 18 %), except for the first 20 s after the presentation of the first sentence (condition, 1; $p = 0.13$, $eta^2 = 7\%$).

The Wilcoxon test within each group showed for normal controls, former schizophrenics, and neurotics a significant increase of the 8- to 13-Hz centroid from baseline to all five conditions (p between 0.05 and 0.005). For acute schizophrenics, however, the reactivity reached significance only in condition 2 (first 20 s after the presentation of the first sentence, $p = 0.05$).

Thus, measured with the centroid, normal controls, former schizophrenics, and neurotics reacted similarly within the alpha band, showing an increase of the centroid value after all stimulus presentations, as compared to the initial resting epoch, in contrast to acute schizophrenics who showed no or very little EEG reactivity.

EEG Reactivity Measured with the Integrated Power

The analysis of variance (fig. 1) showed significant results for all reactivities (p values between 0.09 and 0.001 and eta^2 values between 7 and 18 %).

The Wilcoxon test within each group showed a significant decrease of the 8- to 13-Hz integrated power from initial resting to all five conditions for normal controls and neurotics (p values between 0.10 and 0.01). Acute and former schizophrenics, however, showed no significant changes of the integrated power of the 8- to 13-Hz band.

Thus, measured with the integrated power, normal controls and neurotics reacted similarly within the alpha band, showing a reduction of the power after the stimulus presentation as compared to the resting epoch, in contrast to acute and former schizophrenics who showed no significant group decrease and displayed individual reactivities: in the group of acute schizophrenics 5 subjects reacted with a reduction of alpha power in all five conditions, 5 subjects reacted always with an increase of power, and 12 subjects reacted inconsistently during the experiment. In the group of former schizophrenics 9 subjects reacted always with a reduction of power, 6 subjects always with an increase of power, and 7 subjects inconsistently during the experiment.

Discussion

The results of the study show that there are no statistically significant differences between the mean values of the four groups during the EEG *states of resting* or after presentation of information, as measured with the centroid and the integrated power of the 8- to 13-Hz frequency band. If, however, the EEG reactivity to incoming information, defined as the amount of *change* of the two parameters of the alpha band from the initial resting state to different times after the presentation of the information, is considered, distinct differences between some groups and EEG parameters can be found.

In normals, the information-induced EEG reactivity in the alpha band consists of an increase of the centroid value and a decrease of the integrated power, typical changes which we observed during arousal reactions (orienting responses) in several other studies with normal subjects.

Measured with the centroid normal controls, neurotics and former schizophrenics reacted similarly with a reduction of the alpha band centroid, in contrast to acute schizophrenics who showed no or a very limited reactivity. We have interpreted this finding [*Koukkou,* 1980 a, b, 1982], as an EEG correlate of the productive schizophrenic symptoms which normalize in a good remission. However, measured with the integrated power, former schizophrenics react like acute schizophrenics and different from neurotics and normal controls. Thus, the EEG reactivity differences measured with this parameter are independent of the existence of clinically manifested productive schizophrenic symptoms. These results suggest that measurements of the frequency distribution changes (centroid changes) within the alpha band indicate brain states, and measurements of power changes indicate traits [*Shagass,* 1976] – the different measurements (centroid, power) within the same band having different functional correlations.

We note that the EEG measures in the alpha band did not indicate a deviant EEG state during cognitive processing of information in our drug-free neurotics during the phase of reduction of neurotic symptoms, as compared with normal subjects, although measurements in other EEG bands differentiate normals from symptom-reduced neurotics. This result is in agreement with the report of *Goldstein* [1981] on restoration of statistical features of the EEG of neurotics during epochs of symptom reduction and with the observation that the EEG differences between neurotics and normals subjects relate mainly to the theta and beta band, but not to the alpha band [*Goldstein* et al., 1980, *Hoffmann,* 1980].

Summary

The EEG reactivity to auditory information (the central components of the orienting reaction) was used to examine differences in brain states underlying information processing between neurotics, former schizophrenics, acute schizophrenics, and normal controls. The EEG reactivity was assessed as information-induced changes of two parameters (centroid and integrated power) of the alpha band extracted from power spectral frequency analysis of the EEG. The EEG reactivity of normal controls and neurotics was similar and corresponded to the typical orienting reaction. Acute schizophrenics showed a severely reduced reactivity as measured with both parameters. Former schizophrenics reacted with the centroid like normal controls and neurotics and with the integrated power like acute schizophrenics. These results indicate that within the same frequency band different EEG parameters may have different functional significances.

Acknowledgements

We wish to thank Mr. G. Bomben, Mr. W. Manske and Miss B. Rapp for technical assistance, and Miss B. Kloter for secretarial work.

References

Goldstein, L.: Statistical organizational features of the computerized EEG under various behavioral states. Adv. biol., Psychiat., vol. 6, pp. 12–16 (Karger, Basel 1981).

Goldstein, L.; Denoth, F.; Murri, L.; Stefanini, A.; Muratorio, A.: Automatic computerized analysis of the hemispheric EEG relationships in neurotics and epileptic patients. Adv. biol. Psychiat., vol. 4, pp. 3–13 (Karger, Basel 1980).

Gossop, M.: Theories of neurosis (Springer, Berlin 1981).

Hoffmann, E.: EEG frequency analysis of anxious patients and of normals during resting and during deep muscle relaxation. Adv. biol. Psychiat., vol. 4, pp. 119–130 (Karger, Basel 1980).

Koukkou, M.: EEG correlates of information processing in acute schizophrenics. Adv. biol. Psychiat., vol. 4, pp. 102–110 (Karger, Basel 1980 a).

Koukkou, M.: EEG reactivity in acute schizophrenics reflects deviant (ectropic) state changes during information processing; in Koukkou, Lehmann, Angst, Functional states of the brain: their determinants, pp. 265–290 (Elsevier, Amsterdam 1980 b).

Koukkou, M.: EEG states of the brain, information processing and schizophrenic primary symptoms. Psychiat. Res., pp. 235–244 (Elsevier, Amsterdam 1982).

Lehmann, D.: Fluctuations of functional state: EEG patterns and perceptual and cognitive strategies; in Koukkou, Lehmann, Angst, Functional states of the brain: their determinants, pp. 189–202 (Elsevier, Amsterdam 1980).

Lehmann, D.; Koukkou, M.: Computer analysis of EEG wakefulness sleep patterns during learning of novel and familiar sentences. Electroenceph. clin. Neurophysiol. *37:* 73–84 (1971).

Öhman, A.: The orienting response, attention, and learning: an information-processing perspective; in Kimmel, van Olst, Orlebeke, The orienting reflex in humans, pp. 443–471 (Erlbaum, Hillsdale 1979).
Shagass, Ch.: An electrophysiological view of schizophrenia. Biol. Psychiat. *11:* 3–30 (1976).

M. Koukkou, MD, Research Department, University Hospital of Psychiatry,
CH-8029 Zurich (Switzerland)

Adv. biol. Psychiat, vol. 9, pp. 28–38 (Karger, Basel 1982)

In Quest of the Best Spectral EEG Parameters Towards a Multicentric Consensus for Measuring Normality, Psychopathology and Psychotropic Drug Effects

P. Etevenon[a], *D. Samson-Dollfus*[b], *D. Kemali*[c], *C. Perris*[d 1]

[a] Laboratoire d'EEG Quantitative, Centre Hospitalier Sainte-Anne, Paris, France; [b] Service de Biophysique, Centre Hospitalier Régional et Universitaire de Rouen, Hôpital Charles-Nicolle, Rouen, France; [c] Clinica Psichiatrica, Universita di Napoli, Napoli, Italia; [d] Department of Psychiatry, Umeå Hospital, Umeå, Sweden

«Et vous alors? que cherchez vous»
Le mont analogue, René Daumal

A consensus is growing among the fifty quantitative electroencephalography laboratories operating in the world at the moment. Ten years ago, these laboratories computed electroencephalograms (EEGs), with different techniques, such as integrated amplitude measurement, period analysis, interval analysis, or power spectrum analysis [*Etevenon,* 1977]. At present, the last method encompasses almost all the other methods and, with the advent of mini- and microcomputers with fast Fourier transform micro-programed firmware, spectral analysis has become the most commonly used method of computerized EEG (CEEG) analysis.

However, basic requirements for such a spectral analysis have to be fulfilled. A number of choices have also to be made when different CEEG laboratories are planning to work together. It is necessary to determine the recording conditions, the criteria for choosing the subjects and patients to be recorded, the methods for measuring the effects of drugs and their time courses, and the EEG channels to be recorded.

Multicentric studies appear increasingly necessary in this field of research, not only to augment the number of recorded subjects and patients but also to confirm or refute already available findings on specific charac-

[1] We wish to thank Miss *Lorna Valdés* for translating and typing help. This research was supported by Inserm PRC grant No. 120012 'Santé mentale et cerveau'.

teristics of quantified EEGs in normal controls, and in schizophrenic or depressed patients.

Data can be exchanged between different laboratories in different ways. First, the same subjects can be recorded under the same conditions in different laboratories. Except for the scientist visiting these different places, such an ideal situation is not easily met. However, this procedure is able to reveal differences between equipments and computation techniques. Second, the subjects or patients can be recorded at different locations on magnetic tapes, using similar or compatible frequency modulation (FM) or pulsed code modulation (PCM) magnetic tape recorders. However, such a compatibility is not easy to obtain and often implies having to buy rather expensive tape recorders. Of course, the same tape recorder can be transported to different locations, first for recording purposes and later on for playing back the recorded tapes in another CEEG laboratory. But this is a tedious procedure which is practical only when two or more laboratories are located near each other. A third possibility of exchange is to practice the same EEG analysis, store the results on digital magnetic tapes and mail the tapes between laboratories. However, even to read digital magnetic tapes on different computers is not an easy task. The last and fourth possibility of exchange that we mainly consider in this article, is the use between laboratories of the same computation techniques and then, later on, the exchange of listings made from the same computerized spectral parameters.

Spectral Analysis Requirements

EEG Recording Equipment

The EEG polygraph and the FM or PCM magnetic tape recorder should present less than ± 10° of phase differences between two channels for an EEG frequency range of 0.5–50 Hz. The thermal drive should be less than 2 % in amplitude for 8 h of recording. These technical requirements are necessary for the reliability and replicability of EEG recordings. When recordings have to be made in different laboratories, a similar time constant of, usually, 0.3 s and no filtering have to be used.

Proper Recording Conditions

It is important that the EEG technician should be the same and be trained in handling CEEG equipment in regard to the EEG recordings to be analyzed. The EEG recordings have to be made very carefully with the same electrode positions, low skin resistances (below 5 kΩ) and equivalent resistances between leads. It is better to use small gold-plated electrodes glued on the scalp with special conductive paste.

The rejection of artifacts is very important. It can be done on-line or off-line. In Paris, we use a double rejection technique implemented on-line: a first, predetermined, amplitude threshold followed by a second, manual, delayed rejection. This implies a very fast computer with also an important active memory capacity for temporary buffers. In other laboratories, the rejection is often made off-line after recalling the digitalized epochs of the EEG and looking for the presence of artifacts.

Anti-Aliasing Filters and A/D Conversion

To avoid aliasing errors in power spectrum computation, it is necessary to filter the incoming EEG signals by specially built electronic anti-aliasing filters. In Paris, for instance, with a sampling rate of 200 Hz, we use passive, toroidal, Tchebychef-type filters with a 3-dB cut-off frequency at 62.5 Hz and an attenuation slope of 72 dB per octave. Such filters present 1% amplitude attenuation and a linear phase shift from 0.5 to 82 Hz; above 82 Hz, the attenuation is so important that phase errors may occur. However, Shannons theorem implies that the signal is defined up to 100 Hz only under these conditions, but in the EEG frequency range we may neglect what is above 49 Hz.

The usual calibration of $\pm 50\,\mu V$ must be digitalized as well and taken into consideration for expressing the following sampled EEGs in microvolts. Another digitalized pretreatment of data would be dc removal for obtaining a true zero baseline for every 2.56 second epoch. Similarly, hardware or software digital filtering of lower and higher frequencies should also be used. Similar cut-off frequencies are recommended between laboratories.

Fast Fourier Transform Analysis

The sampling rate is usually determined together with the time resolution or the frequency resolution, depending on the duration of the epoch chosen and the number of points defined in one operating block. In Paris, a sampling rate of 200 Hz is chosen with a 0.39 Hz frequency resolution for epochs of 2.56 s defined for blocks of 512 digitalized points.

The total duration of the EEG recording is 5 min, free of artifacts. This means that 120 epochs of 2.56 s are computed and subjected to spectral analysis. The coefficient of variation being then less than 10 % statistical stability is warranted despite possible non-stationarity of the EEG signals, which appears to be less important than stability [*Etevenon,* 1977].

An error of computation in fast Fourier transform (FFT) analysis is called the Gibbs or rectangular window error. In order to minimize this computational error we generally multiply the digitalized EEG signals of each epoch with a so-called cosine tapper or a bell-shaped time curve used as a filter. In Paris, this filter, applied in the time domain, is a microprogramed Hanning window.

Finally, if we want to express the power spectrum computed after complex multiplication of the FFT, in microwatts and not only in arbitrary units, we have to use a multiplicative calibration constant applied to every value of the FFT. In Paris the constant chosen is 51,200 and equals $2\times4\times(50\times50)/(\text{frequency resolution} = 0.39)$. The first factor, 2, is produced by the fact that half of the FFT is usually computed, the second factor, 4, is a correction factor for the attenuation of the Hanning window, the third factor is the squared 50 μV calibration signal already taken into account. After using this calibration multiplicative constant, the computed power spectra are expressed in true absolute values and their square roots are expressed in absolute root mean square (RMS) amplitude microvolt values.

Spectral Analysis

Averaged power spectra over 5 min of EEG recording can be computed for every EEG channel after computation of evolutive power spectra (which are equivalent to the compressed spectral array of Bickford). This can be followed by further statistical spectral analysis comparing EEG recordings within or between subjects, applying spectral t tests [*Etevenon,* 1978; *Etevenon* et al., 1978, 1979a, b], analysis of variance [*Kemali* et al., 1980] and nonparametric tests [*Samson-Dollfus,* 1979].

Spectral Parameters

After computing a large number of spectral parameters from the evolutive power spectra and the averaged power spectra, we applied multivariate statistical spectral analysis together with step-by-step discriminant and regression analyses to a large number of quantified EEGs. As a result we were able to observe a great redundancy between EEG spectral parameters. The principal types of parameters which appear to be the best descriptors of the quantified EEGs and which also present the least redundancy between them are: the mean frequencies, computed by the centroid formula; the RMS absolute amplitude values, expressed in microvolts; the RMS relative amplitude percentages, analogous to time percentages; the ratios computed for one of these parameters, between EEG channels (right/left, anterior/posterior areas), between frequency bands (like alpha/theta ratio which is a good indicator of drowsiness). These four types of parameters also present standard errors, variances and coefficients of variation which can be computed from the successive evolutive power spectra. This computation doubles the amount of parameters but provides dispersion values for these basic parameters. Further statistics on these dispersion values would be better computed using nonparametric tests instead of the more classical parametric tests.

Moreover, such parameters have to be computed not only for the total raw EEGs but also for each of the EEG frequency bands: delta, theta, alpha, beta. We will later discuss the critical choice of such frequency bands.

Of course, other parameters can be computed as well. This is, for instance, the case of coherences and phase spectra between two EEG channels. New problems then arise, for example, what would be the proper statistics to apply to such complex parameters. How could we assert the influence of other EEG channels if we do not compute still more refined and sophisticated parameters such as residual power spectra and multiple coherences [*Etevenon,* 1978]?

Multivariate Statistical Analysis

After data reduction and computation of the characteristic spectral parameters quantifying EEGs, multivariate statistical analysis of the data is generally performed in a computer center. Correspondence analysis or factorial analysis can be made between EEGs, where each EEG is considered as a vector consisting of an array of a descriptive set of parameters. This analysis can also be applied to parameters where each parameter is an array composed of the specific values taken for each different EEG. By cluster analysis, subgroups can be determined from the data. For instance, hierarchical arborescent classification analysis of quantified EEGs provides subgroups which can be compared with clinical populations. Discriminant analysis applied to the set of data already classified according to clinical populations or subtypes provides the parameters which are the best descriptors of the populations. What are the sensitivity and the predictability of such a step-by-step discrimination? We prefer using a quadratic discriminant algorithm instead of a linear technique which is less powerful in discriminating between the data. Finally, multiple covariance analysis may be used to compare the same EEGs by different quantification methods. It is obvious that such sophisticated statistical analyses are tedious, time-consuming, and also very expensive in terms of running time of large computers. When data are obtained in a multicentric study, the same statistical procedure should be applied to the set of data by a good team of experienced statisticians.

As examples, *Etevenon* et al. [1979a, b; 1981] have been able, using these techniques, to separate two populations of EEGs of normal volunteers (characterized by high or a low alpha amplitude), two populations of EEGs of schizophrenic patients (deficiency patients or productive paranoid patients), and one small population of EEGs of chronic nonschizophrenic patients (very hypovariable hig alpha amplitude). When considering the parameters instead of the EEGs, all the different frequency bands were well discriminated by the RMS amplitude parameter in the first factorial plane, especially the alpha amplitude, which was very different from the delta, theta and beta amplitudes. The mean frequency parameter was a similarly good descriptor, discriminating the different frequency bands. However, the dispersion parameters around these RMS amplitudes or mean frequencies were less powerful after principal component analysis. The different frequency bands were often centered in the factorial planes and overlapped each other.

Samson-Dollfus et al. [1978] have also discriminated subgroups of EEGs of patients and normal volunteers by the age factor. *Kemali* et al. (this volume) have recently compared diagnoses and CEEGs from Italy and Sweden using multivariate analyses.

Hierarchy of Changes

Under this title we present the hierarchy, the branched tree, the basic rules of the CEEG method.

Parameters and Frequency Bands

We have already presented the EEG parameters. It is trivial to say that an RMS amplitude is not a mean frequency and that a position parameter is not a dispersion parameter. This is why, in the space of parameters defined by arrays of EEG values, multivariate analysis is separating first between parameters. Nevertheless, for a specific CEEG study it is very important to choose a proper set of parameters. For instance, *Etevenon* in Paris and also *Matousek* in Göteborg (this volume) prefer to use RMS amplitudes expressed both in true absolute values and in percentages instead of power values, the square root reduces the variance of the power values, and the RMS amplitudes expressed in microvolts are well understood by clinicians. But looking for hemispheric brain lateralization, *Goldstein* (this volume) and *d'Elia and Perris* [1977] preferred using variances around amplitudes, despite the fact that these values were not normally distributed, which imposed the choice of nonparametric statistics.

Now, frequency limits have to be very well defined. If they changed between laboratories, the same parameter might present different values. For instance, the alpha range was first considered as a broad band between 7.4 and 13 Hz [*Itil,* 1979; *Etevenon,* 1978]. A finer band between 8.5 and 12.5 appears to be a better choice, and even *Matousek* in Sweden and *Herrmann* in Berlin are splitting this alpha band into a low alpha-1 (8.5–10.5 Hz) and a high alpha-2 band (10.5–12.5 Hz). These two alpha bands apparently exhibit an inverse behavior: after amphetamine administration, the alpha-1 band increases in intensity whereas the alpha-2 band decreases; as a consequence, the broader alpha band does not change. Confronted with this problem in multicentric studies, the involved laboratories must agree on almost similar limits for the frequency bands. *Koukkou-Lehmann* (this volume) has used programs with variable frequency bands, which is a possible solution to this problem.

Recording Conditions and Modalities

Shagass (this volume) presents the different modalities which are the first choices in CEEG or evoked-potential studies. The recording conditions have to be specified at first. The spontaneous EEG may be recorded with closed or open eyes, in a free vigilance situation or in a controlled vigilance situation avoiding drowsiness. Hyperventilation and photic stimulation can also be chosen as recording conditions.

Populations

The recorded subjects or patients should be selected from homogeneous populations. However, such a homogeneity is rare and is generally obtained after statistical multivariate analysis of CEEGs. For example, among a population of quantified EEGs recorded from normal volunteers, two subgroups have been found: a high-alpha and a low-alpha subgroup [*Etevenon,* 1978]. Similarly, a population of schizophrenic patients has been classified according to clinical criteria into three classes: 'residual' deficient, 'paranoid' productive patients and a mixed group called 'others'. After statistical analysis, these classes have been found to be different from each other when considering some specific spectral parameters [*Etevenon* et al., 1979a, 1981]. Another classification of such patients is obtained when considering drug responders and nonresponders. The age of the subjects is also very important. EEG subtypes have been found by *Samson-Dollfus* et al. [1979], separating young from adult and elderly people. *d'Elia and Perris* [1977] have also differentiated the EEGs of depressed patients from other groups by considering right versus left within amplitude variance measurements.

Drug Effects versus Placebo

CEEG has been used preferentially for the past 20 years in order to assess the specific effects of psychotropic drugs on the EEG. *Fink* et al. have described specific psychotropic 'profiles' whereas *Goldstein* et al. published several reports on the effects of various drugs in different homogeneous populations of controls and patients. Usually, placebo responders are excluded from small sample studies. However, it appears that intrasubject variability between placebo recordings is not too high [*Etevenon* et al., 1981]. This variability factor could be used as a test of the homogeneity of successive recordings within subjects.

Not only do different drugs present different profiles, but also the same drug may have different effects in the same population when considering the time courses, the acute or chronic administration, the dose-response curve, the route and rate of administration, and the galenic form. Therefore, pharmacokinetics can be measured together with CEEG, allowing biovailability studies.

EEG Channels

The last changes to be observed after proper setting of the preceding factors are functional bioelectrical activities which may differ from one EEG channel to another. We have already mentioned the lateralization changes between the right and left hemispheres which were different in depressed and i schizophrenic patients [*d'Elia and Perris,* 1977; *Etevenon* et al., 1979b; *Flor-Henry,* this volume; *Kemali* et al., 1980].

Two problems occur. The first one is the choice of the position of the electrodes. Frontal electrodes are often contaminated by ocular movements and muscle ativity. Occipital electrodes are less contaminated by artifacts and present usually greater amplitudes but may be less sensitive to drug effects. The second problem that arises is the choice of the electrode setting (bipolar or unipolar) and also of the reference electrode: earlobes, vertex, forehead, or chin, or also a common averaged electrode. In Paris, we use bipolar electrodes, usually right and left centroparietal and parieto-occipital electrodes, but we also record with fronto-temporal electrodes when it is possible.

Discussion

A number of choices remain to be made: the choice of the time window, usually 2.56 s. However, to achieve a greater stationarity of the EEG epochs, some scientists prefer 5.12- or better 10.24-second epochs. But the latter choice implies a smaller number of averaged epochs, and this means a greater statistical variability. For practical reasons and from our experience with cmposite spectra, we prefer using 2.56-second epochs and averaging 120 of these epochs. This means to record 5-min EEGs which may cause drowsiness in the subject, but less than 5 min may be statistically too variable. We have also used a sampling rate of 200 Hz and a frequency resolution of 0.4 Hz. Of course, when the frequency resolution is smaller than 0.4 Hz, computation of mean frequencies with the centroid formula [*Lehmann and Koukkou,* 1980] is more accurate, but the variability of adjacent frequency points also increases.

A second type of choice is to select the limits of the spectral frequency bands and also to select the position of the EEG channels to be recorded. One of the best choices of frequency limits, following the work of *Kubicki* et al. [1979] is: delta from 1.5 to 6 Hz; theta from 6 to 8.5 Hz; alpha-1 from 8.5 to 10.5 Hz; alpha-2 from 10.5 to 12.5 Hz; beta-1 from 12.5 to 18.5 Hz; beta-2 from 18.5 to 21 Hz and beta-3 from 21 to 30 Hz. The choice of the EEG channels depends on the study to be made and also on the equipment of the CEEG laboratory. Except for pharmacological studies in which *Fink and Itil,* for example, record only one channel (Cz-02), we prefer recording at least four EEG channels. A new research of great interest is the topographical mapping of spectral activities or evoked-potential activities simultaneously recorded over 16 EEG channels (*Buchsbaum,* this volume).

A third type of choice is the appraisal of clinical symptoms or psychological testing. This is the well-known problem of nosography.

After exposing these open problems and trying to present some practical solutions for reaching a basic consensus and the compatibility required by multicentric and multidisciplinary studies, we may compare our CEEG field of research with similar ones in geophysics, astrophysics and meteorology. These earth and sky sciences are heavily dependent on applied mathematics, i. e. data analysis, informatics, but also on fundamental theoretical physics, like potential theory and tensor algebra. The meteorologist is able to predict cyclones, perhaps the computerized electroencephalographist will be able to predict in a near future, not only already assessed psychotropic drug profiles, but also pathological diagnoses and their changes following drug treatments. This is still research and development in the blue sky.

References

Elia, G. d'; Jacobsson, L.; Knorring, L. von; Matisson B.; Mjorndal, T.; Oreland, I.: Changes in psychopathology in relation to EEG variables and visual averaged evoked responses (V.AER) in schizophrenic patients treated with penfluridol or thiothixene. Acta psychiat. scand. *55:* 309–318 (1977).

Etevenon, P.: Etude méthodologique de l'électroencéphalographie quantitative. Application à quelques exemples; thèse D. Sc., Paris VI (Copédith, Paris 1978).

Etevenon, P.; Pidoux, B.: From biparametric to multidimensional analysis of EEG; in Remond, EEG informatics. A didactic review of methods and applications of EEG data processing, pp. 193–214 (Elsevier, Amsterdam 1977).

Etevenon, P.; Pidoux, B.: Progresses of statistical spectral analysis in pharmacoelectroencephalography. Pharmakopsychiatr. Neuro-Psychopharmakol. *12:* 102–110 (1979).

Etevenon, P.; Pidoux, B.; Peron-Magnan, P.; Rioux, P.; Verdeaux, G.; Boissier, J.R.; Deniker, P.: Electroencephalography statistical spectral analysis and new trends of quantitative electroencephalography; in Deniker, Radoucos-Thomas, Villeneuve, Neuropsychopharmacology, pp. 1141–1150 (Pergamon Press, Oxford 1978).

Etevenon, P.; Pidoux, B.; Rioux, P.: Strategy of statistical spectral analysis in drug studies. A methological synopsis; in Saletu, Neuropsychopharmacology, pp. 383–391 (Pergamon Press, Oxford 1979a).

Etevenon, P.; Pidoux, B.; Rioux, P.; Peron-Magnan, P.; Verdeaux, G.; Deniker, P.: Intra- and interhemispheric EEG differences quantified by spectral analysis. Acta psychiat. scand. *60:* 57–68 (1979b).

Etevenon, P.; Pidoux, B.; Cottereau, M.J.; Peron-Magnan, P.; Zarifian, E.; Verdeaux, G.; Deniker, P.: Quantitative EEG analysis of high-dosage haloperidol effects in therapy-resistant schizophrenic patients. Adv. biol. Psychiat., vol. 4, pp. 175–187 (Karger, Basel 1980).

Etevenon, P.; Peron-Magnan, P.; Rioux, P.; Pidoux, B.; Bisserbe, J.C.; Verdeaux, G.; Deniker, P.: Schizophrenia assessed by computerized EEG. Adv. biol. Psychiat., vol. 6, pp. 29–34 (Karger, Basel 1981).

Feighner, J.P.; Robins, E.; Guze, S.B.; Woodruff, R.A.; Winokur, G.; Munoz, R.: Diagnostic criteria for use in psychiatric research. Archs gen. Psychiat. *26:* 57–63 (1972).

Fink, M.; Itil, T.M.; Clyde, D.: The classification of psychoses by quantitative EEG measures; in Wortis, Recent advances in biological psychiatry, vol. 8, pp. 305–312 (Plenum Press, New York 1966).

Flor-Henry, P.: Lateralized temporal-limbic dysfunction and psychopathology. Ann. N.Y. Acad. Sci. *280:* 777–795 (1976).

Flor-Henry, P.; Koles, Z.J.: EEG studies in depression, mania and normals: evidence for partial shifts of laterality in the affective psychoses. Adv. biol. Psychiat., vol. 4, pp. 21–43 (Karger, Basel 1980).

Goldstein, L.; Sugerman, A.A.; Stolberg, H.; Murphee, H.B.; Pfeiffer, C.C.: Electro-cerebral activity in schizophrenics and non-psychotic subjects. Quantitative EEG amplitude analysis. Electroenceph. clin. Neurophysiol. *19:* 350–361 (1965).

Itil, T.M.: Qualitative and quantitative EEG findings in schizophrenia. Schizophrenia Bull. *3:* 61–78 (1977).

Itil, T.M.; Saletu, B.; Davis, S.: EEG findings in chronic schizophrenics based on digital computer period analysis and analog power spectra. Biol. Psychiat. *5/1* (1972).

Kemali, D.; Vacca, L.; Nolfe, G.; Iorio, G.; De Carlo, R.: Hemispheric EEG quantitative asymmetries in schizophrenics and depressed patients. Adv. biol. Psychiat., vol. 4, pp. 14–20 (Karger, Basel 1980).

Kubicki, S.; Herrmann, W.M.; Fichte, K.; Freund, G.: Reflections on the topics: EEG frequency bands and regulation of vigilance. Pharmakopsychiat. Neuro-Psychopharmakol. *12:* 237–245 (1979).

Lehmann, D.; Koukkou, M.: Classes of spontaneous, private experiences and human background EEG; in Pfurtscheller et al., Event-related rhytmic cortical activities; behavioral correlates (Elsevier, Amsterdam 1980).

Lifshitz, K.; Gradijan, J.: Relationships between measures of the coefficient of variation of the mean absolute EEG voltage and spectral intensities in schizophrenic and control subjects. Biol. Psychiat. *5:* 149–163 (1972).

Lifshitz, K.; Gradijan, J.: Spectral evaluation of the electroencephalogram: power and variability in chronic schizophrenics and control subjects. Psychophysiology *11:* 479–490 (1974).

Marjerrisson, G.; Krause, A.E.; Keogh, R.P.: Variability of the EEG in schizophrenia quantitative analysis with a modulus voltage integrator. Electroenceph. Clin. Neurophysiol. *24:* 35–41 (1968).

Pidoux, B.; Peron-Magnan, P.; Etevenon, P.; Verdeaux, G.; Deniker, P.: L'activité alpha dans un groupe de schizophrènes: analyse spectrale et comparaison avec un groupe témoin. Rev. Electroencéphalogr. clin. Neurophysiol. *8:* 283–293 (1978).

Samson-Dollfus, D.; Rogler, M.; Souliac, B.: Application de l'analyse spectrale de l'EEG à l'étude des malades atteints d'insuffisance vasculaire cérébrale. Rev. Electroencéphalogr. clin. Neurophysiol. *6:* 328–329 (1976).

P. Etevenon, Inserm, 2, rue d'Alésia, F-75014 Paris (France)

Adv. biol. Psychiat., vol. 9, pp. 39–43 (Karger, Basel 1982)

Ischemic Pain Stress: Effect on Lateralization of EEG Amplitudes

Cary L. Hamlin, Leonide Goldstein[1]

CMDNJ-Rutgers Medical School, Piscataway, N.J., USA

Introduction

The cerebral mechanisms involved in the perception and sensation of pain have been of great interest to a large number of investigators for a long time [for review see *Beecher,* 1957]. The development of computerized EEG analysis methods, which enable the determination of the relative state of activation of one or the other hemisphere, has opened new research possibilities, including the objective determination of the nature of the feelings and sensations associated with pain. Thus, relative activation of the left hemisphere can indicate a verbal-rational handling of the sensory information while a relative activation of the right hemisphere would tend to suggest the enhancement of the affective-emotional activities [*Flor-Henry,* 1979; *Goldstein,* 1979].

In a first study involving hemispheric EEG recordings during experimental pain induction, it was found that cold pressure produced a contralateral activation which was abolished following induction of hypnotic analgesia, at least in highly hypnotizable subjects [*Karlin* et al., 1980]. However, since it has been argued that cold pressor pain is not comparable to clinical pain, it was decided to investigate this problem using a prodecure recognized as being more relevant to clinical pain: ischemic muscular pain [*Smith* et al., 1966; *McGlashan* et al., 1969].

[1] The excellent assistance of *Natalia Krawciw* and *Albert Jekelis* is gratefully acknowledged.

Methods

Subjects and Recording Procedures

The subjects were 10 adult, right-handed male subjects (mean age: 29; range 22–38), in good physical health. The experiments took place in a dimly lit, sound-attenuated room, where the subjects were comfortably seated. They were alone during the baselines; however, during the sequences involving pain, one of the experimenters was present in the room in order to manipulate the instrumentation.

The sessions involved six segments. First, there was a 5-min baseline recording with no instructions given except the suggestion of as much relaxation as possible. This was followed by inflation up to 200 mm Hg of a sphygmomanometer cuff placed on one of the arms. The pressure was maintained during 5 min. Moreover, during the first 90 s, there was also isometric muscle contraction of 100 mm Hg over the area of the hand of the arm on which ischemic pain was produced. Following deflection of the cuff, there was a 3-min recording of the 'recovery from pain'. This was followed by a 30-min rest during which the subjects were asked to rate the severity of pain on a 0 to 10 (maximal) scale, giving values for the first 90 s and the end of the 5-min ischemia. The same procedure was repeated, using the contralateral arm and hand. The order of right and left arms being first and second was alternated between subjects.

EEG Recording and Analytical Procedures

The EEG was recorded from the right and left temporal leads (T4-T3) with Cz as common reference and the middle forehead for grounding. Besides direct ink tracings, the signals were digitalized on-line by analog integration, for all frequencies between 1.3 and 30 Hz (total power$^{1/2}$), for successive epochs of 5-second duration. There were approximately 60 epochs for the baselines and the same number for the pain segments. The data were stored on floppy disks and analyzed off-line with a 6800-based Southwest Technical Products Macrocomputer, using a program which estimated the following parameters separately for each segment: (1) the means and variances of the distribution of amplitudes and (2) a chronogram of the interrelationships of amplitudes between right and left temporals based on on the differences between the values of the right/left ratio for each epoch and the overall global ratio across conditions. This enabled the computation of the proportion of time with relative activation in one or the other hemisphere for the baselines and the pain segments.

The procedures were carefully explained to the subjects before the sessions. They signed a consent form.

Results

Subjective Reports of the Severity of Ischemic Pain

There were no statistically significant differences in the scores of severity of ischemic pain when the right or left arms and hands were used. However, this was not the case for the first and second pain segments. For the initial 90 s, the values were 5.5 ± 1.6 and 4.2 ± 1.5, respectively, and for the end of the pain segments 6.0 ± 2.2 and 4.8 ± 2.0, respectively. The one-tailed t test yields a $p \leq 0.05$ for both differences.

Table I. % time (± SE) with relatively higher or lower activity in the right temporal

Baseline I	Pain on R	Pain on L	Baseline II	Pain on R	Pain on L
Whole group of subjects					
55.5 ± 5.4 (n = 10)	58.2 ± 6.6 (n = 6)	54.7 ± 10.6	49.6 ± 6.1 (n = 10)	50.2 ± 12.0 (n = 4)	53.2 ± 5.1 (n = 6)
Subjects with activation on the R during the baselines					
70.0 ± 1.5[1] (n = 9)	35.0 ± 9.8* (n = 3)	47.0 ± 6.5* (n = 6)			
Subjects with activation on the L during the baselines					
38.3 ± 3.0[2] (n = 11)	63.6 ± 4.8* (n = 7)	64.0 ± 3.9* (n = 4)			

R = Right; L = Left.
* Statistically significant difference with baseline t = 4.8 add 5.8, respectively, $p < 0.001$.
[1] 71.2 ± 2.2 for the first baseline and 68.5 ± 1.9 for the second baseline.
[2] 39.8 ± 2.2 for the first baseline and 37.0 ± 5.5 for the second baseline.

Percent Time with Relative Activation in the Right and/or Left Hemispheres

The data are listed in table I. As can be seen, when averages are made across the whole group of subjects, it does not appear that any change in relation to baselines occurs when the subjects experience ischemic pain in either of the arms. None of the differences are statistically significant.

However, if one groups the subjects who happened to have activation in the right temporal during baseline, it appears that ischemic pain, regardless of the arm used, produces a marked, highly statistically significant shift of the activation to the left temporal. The reverse occurs when the baseline reveals left temporal activation: in this case it is the right which is activated during ischemic pain, again regardless of the arm on which the cuff was placed. The averaging of the values during the first and second baselines is justified by a lack of significant differences between them, as mentioned in table I.

Discussion

The effect of ischemic pain on cerebral laterality of the EEG has not been investigated thus far. Unlike verbal-analytical or visual-spatial stimuli which have been found to produce activation of the left and right temporals, respectively [*Goldstein,* 1979], ischemic pain stimulation does not produce such specific effects, regardless of its point of origin. However, our data suggest that it does produce a consistent effect upon EEG lateralization which is that it reverses the prevailing state before its imposition.

It is to be emphasized that this pre-pain state is different from what is commonly found in normal subjects without impending stress. Instead of a range of 45–55 % time spontaneous activation in one or the other hemispheres [*Goldstein,* 1979, 1980], one finds, in the case of impending ischemic pain, activations ranging from 60 to 80 % time in one or the other temporal. While the meaning of this finding awaits further experimentation, an attractive hypothesis is that it corresponds to coping strategies which are developed during the baselines. From the reports obtained from the subjects, it can be seen how differently they approached the impending stress. Some diverted their thoughts to self-generation of music tunes or careful examination of the wall they were facing; others attempted to analyze and anticipate the features of the upcoming stress. Unfortunately, one cannot rate these reports in a way which would permit their comparison directly with EEG data.

In spite of subjective reports of lesser pain during the second sequence by comparison with the first, there was no detectable differences in EEG measures. This might be due to the apparent insensitivity of the EEG measures to denote relatively small-scale changes.

If one defines a marked decrease in the percent time activation as a 'disruption', one can seek an explanation for the shift of the prevailing EEG lateralization during pain as resulting from one of the following: (a) disruption of the ipsilateral activity without change of the activity of the contralateral temporal; (b) activity of the ipsilateral disrupted and that of the contralateral increased; (c) activities of both ipsilateral and contralateral disrupted, but one more than the other; (d) activity of the ipsilateral unchanged and that of the contralateral increased; (e) activities of both sides increased but that of the contralateral to a larger extent.

Further experimentation will be needed in order to select which of these mechanisms best fits the data.

Summary

10 normal, male subjects were exposed to 5 min of ischemic pain on each arm in succession. The effects upon the lateralization of the EEG from the temporals were analyzed by comparing the pre-pain to pain conditions. It was found that ischemic pain produced a marked, highly significant, reversal of lateralized activation, regardless of the hemisphere where it prevailed before and regardless of the arm upon which the pain was imposed.

References

Beecher, H. K.: The measurement of pain. Prototype for the quantitative study of subjective responses. Pharmac. Rev.. *9:* 59–209 (1957).

Flor-Henry, P.: On certain aspects of the localization of the cerebral system regulating and determining emotion. Biol. Psychiat. *14:* 677–698 (1979).

Goldstein, L.: Some relationships between quantified hemispheric EEG and behavioral states in man; in Gruzelier, Flor-Henry, Hemispheric asymmetries of function in psychopathology, pp. 237–254 (Elsevier/North Holland Biomedical Press, Amsterdam 1979).

Goldstein, L.: Is cerebral laterality a myth? Res. Commun. psychol. psychiat. Behav. *5:* 291–301 (1980).

Karlin, R.; Morgan, D.; Goldstein, L.: Hypnotic analgesia: a preliminary investigation of quantitated hemispheric electroencephalographic and attentional correlates. J. abnorm. soc. Psychol. *89:* 591–594 (1980).

McGlashan, T. H.; Evans, F. J.; Orne, M. T.: The nature of hypnotic analgesia and placebo response to experimental pain. Psychosom. Med. *31:* 227–246 (1969).

Smith, G. M.; Egbert, L. D.; Markowitz, R. A.; Mosteller, F.; Beecher, H. K.: An experimental pain method sensitive to morphine in man: the submaximum effort tourniquet technique. J. Pharmac. exp. Ther. *154:* 324–332 (1966).

C. L. Hamlin, MD, CMDNJ-Rutgers Medical School, Piscataway, NJ 08854 (USA)

Adv. biol. Psychiat., vol. 9, pp. 44–49 (Karger, Basel 1982)

Psychiatric Diagnostic Correlates of Evoked Potential Topographic Factors[1]

Charles Shagass, Richard A. Roemer, John J. Straumanis, Jr.[2]

Temple University Medical School and Eastern Pennsylvania Psychiatric Institute Philadelphia, Pa., USA

Previous reports of results obtained with our comprehensive evoked potential (EP) recording procedure have dealt with comparisons between major psychoses, nonpsychotic psychiatric conditions, and normals with respect to general waveshape characteristics [*Shagass* et al., 1977, 1978b], topography of EP peaks [*Shagass* et al., 1979a, 1980a], and waveshape stability in time [*Shagass* et al., 1979b]. While EP characteristics, including the topography of certain components, were found deviant from normal in patients with major psychoses, there were almost no significant deviations in nonpsychotics. This paper presents evidence that EP characteristics of neurotics do differ from normal, but that the deviations are unlike those of chronic schizophrenics. The subject samples are considerably larger than in previous reports. Also, we have employed a different approach to EP topographic analysis, which involves factor analysis of automatically obtained amplitude measures.

Methods

The EP recording procedure has been described previously [*Shagass* et al., 1977, 1978b]. Briefly, EPs were recorded from 14 scalp leads and one eye monitor lead (EOG) referenced to linked ears. Randomly intermingled stimuli included left and right median nerve shocks for somatosensory EPs, designated as LSEP and RSEP, respectively, checkerboard pattern flashes to elicit visual EPs (VEPs), and binaural clicks for auditory EPs (AEPs). Each EP (512 data points, 1-ms sampling) was the average of 192 sweeps.

[1] Research supported (in part) by USPHS grant MH 12507.

[2] We thank the following for their assistance: *I. C. Hung, J. Kline, M. Kormanik, A. McGrath, W. Nixon* and *S. Slepner*.

The average deviation amplitude measure [*Shagass,* 1972] was obtained by computing the mean deviation of the data points in an epoch from the epoch mean, disregarding sign. Average deviations were computed for six overapping epochs as follows: SEPs – 15–30, 15–49, 31–99, 50–199, 100–299, 200–450 ms; VEPs – 50–129, 75–129, 120–249, 75–249, 129–249, 75–450 ms; AEPs – 15–49, 40–99, 40–139, 100–239, 140–239, 40–450 ms. Before factor analysis, the scalp lead average deviations were adjusted for their regression upon the corresponding epoch average deviations in the EOG recording. The EPs for a total sample of acceptable first run tests on 253 patients and 99 nonpatient controls were used for this adjustment and the subsequent factor analyses. Principal components analysis with varimax rotation was applied to the adjusted average deviations across 14 leads. For the 24 factor analyses, the solutions yielded two factors in 15 instances, three factors in 8, and a single factor in one, accounting for 73–85 % of the variance. Factors were interpreted topographically by determining the leads at which factor loadings exceeded 0.400; the early epoch SEP factors suggested greater activity in the hemisphere ipsilateral or contralateral to the stimulus, but most factors reflected either anterior or posterior lead preponderance.

Factor scores were computed for all subjects, and those for subjects in age and sex matched diagnostic groups were compared by multivariate (Manova) profile analysis [*Morrison,* 1967], and also by a conservative analysis of variance (Anova). Present data are for two comparisons: (1) chronic schizophrenics (21 paranoid, 24 undifferentiated, 1 simple), nonpsychotic patients (30 neuroses, 16 personality disorders) and nonpatient controls (15 females, 31 males; median age, 26), and (2) neuroses and controls (42 each, 21 females, 21 males; median age, 30). Diagnoses, made independently by two senior psychiatrists, agreed with the relevant *Feighner* et al. [1972] research diagnostic criteria in nearly all cases. We attempted to test patients after at least 7 days free of medication; the actual interval ranged from 3 days to an indefinite interval greater than 100 days (median, 10 days).

Results

Chronic Schizophrenics vs. Nonpsychotics vs. Controls

The analyses for 24 epochs yielded 20 Manovas, 15 parallelism tests (profiles), 10 Anovas, and 10 interactions significant at $p < 0.05$. Analyses utilizing factor scores for all six epochs gave significant Manovas and profiles for LSEP, RSEP and AEP, and a significant interaction for VEP. The general pattern of the results can be seen in figure 1, which displays mean amplitude factor scores for epochs with minimum overlap. For LSEP and RSEP, both schizophrenics and nonpsychotics had higher early epoch amplitudes than controls; the differentiating factor scores reflected ipsilateral hemisphere activity. Late epoch SEP amplitudes were lowest in schizophrenics, intermediate in controls, and highest in nonpsychotics; both anterior and posterior factors were involved. VEP amplitudes were almost the same in schizophrenics and controls, and lower than those of nonpsychotics for three posterior factors. For the 40–99 ms AEP epoch, a

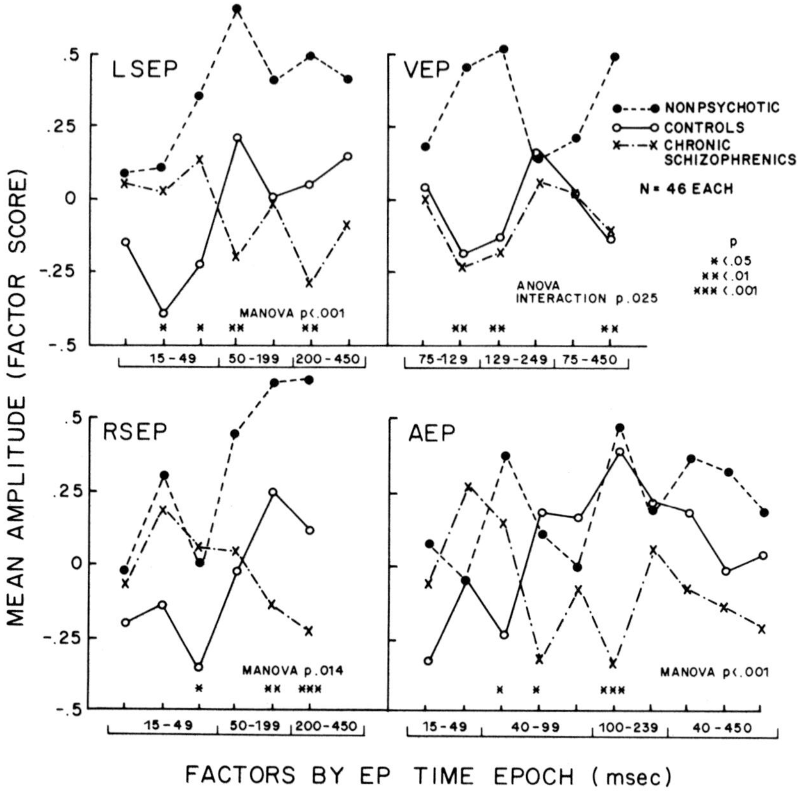

Fig. 1. Amplitudes expressed as topographic factor scores based on average deviation measures for epochs with minimal overlap. Data for age and sex matched chronic schizophrenics, nonpsychotics, and nonpatient controls (n = 46 each), Manova and Anova statements based on analyses including all factors for 6 epochs; p values show significant univariate effects.

posterior factor score was higher for both patient groups than for controls, while a central factor score was lower for the schizophrenics than for the other groups. The schizophrenics were also significantly lower than nonpsychotics or controls with respect to an anterior factor in the 100–239 ms epoch, and lower generally.

Neuroses vs. Controls

The analyses for six epochs gave differences for the first three SEP epochs, the last four VEP epochs, and the 40–99 ms AEP epoch. Figure 2

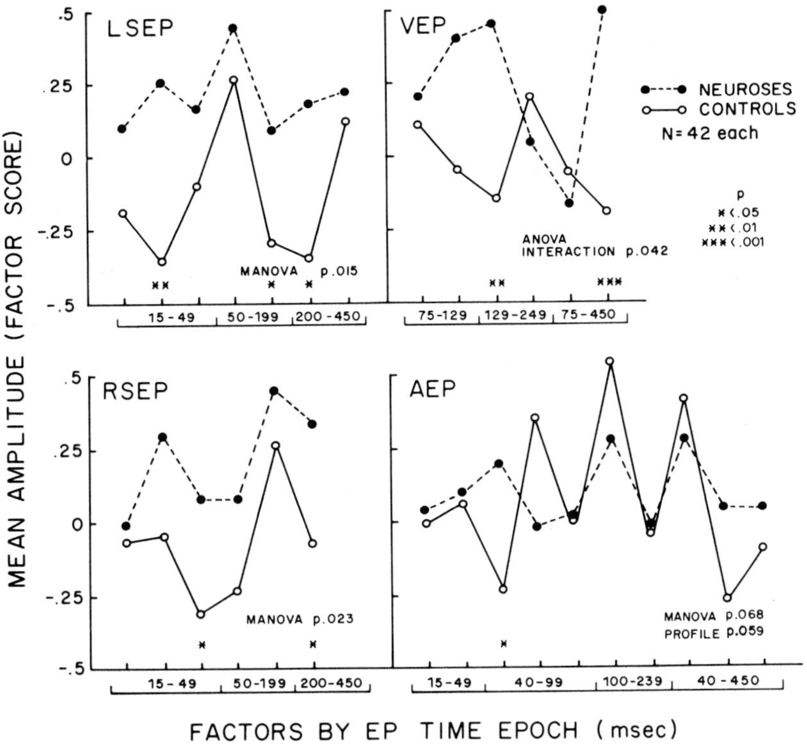

Fig. 2. Amplitude factor scores for 42 neurotics and 42 controls of same age and sex. Arrangements as in figure 1.

shows the results for minimally overlapping epochs. Since 30 of the 42 neurotic patients were included among the 46 nonpsychotics of figure 1, the similarities between the groups are to be expected. The significant differences for the early SEP epoch reflected ipsilateral factors and all other differences involved posterior factors.

Discussion

Present results for chronic schizophrenics seem to be concordant with previous EP findings showing that they have higher early epoch and lower later epoch SEP amplitudes than normals and also lower AEP amplitudes after 100 ms [*Shagass*, et al., 1978a]. The greater than normal early AEP amplitude (posterior leads) of schizophrenics is a new finding emerging from the factor analysis separation of anterior and posterior activity. Also new is the evidence that early epoch SEP amplitude is greater mainly in recordings from the ipsilateral hemisphere in both schizophrenics and neurotics; the finding suggests that some mechanism that normally limits ipsilateral hemisphere discharge may be impaired in these conditions.

It should be noted that our neurotic group contained only 'dysthymic' disorders, since none were hysteric, and that the results were about the same for anxiety, depressive and obsessive-compulsive neuroses. Greater than normal VEP amplitude in dysthymic neuroses has been reported once [*Shagass and Schwartz,* 1965], but other EP findings in neuroses have been either normal or deviant in the same direction as psychoses [*Shagass* et al., 1978a]. Present evidence that EP characteristics of neurotics deviate from normal in a direction opposite to that of schizophrenics represents a new finding with encouraging implications for future applications of EP measurements to differential diagnosis. In particular, the patterning of the differences with respect to early and late EP events, sensory modality (fig. 1), and their anteroposterior distribution suggests considerable diagnostic specificity.

Summary

Somatosensory, visual and auditory evoked potentials (EPs) were recorded from 14 scalp leads and an eye monitor (EOG) lead in 352 subjects. Automatic (average deviation) amplitude measurements for the scalp lead EPs, adjusted for their correlations with EOG activity, were factor analyzed across leads. The resulting topographically interpretable factor scores were used to compare the following age- and sex-matched groups: (1) chronic schizophrenics, nonpsychotics and controls (46 each), and (2) neurotics and controls (42 each). EP factor scores of both neurotics and chronic schizophrenics deviated from normal, but in different ways.

References

Feighner, J.P.; Robins, E.; Guze, S.B.; Woodruff, R.A.; Winokur, G.; Munoz, R.: Diagnostic criteria for use in psychiatric research. Archs gen. Psychiat. *26:* 57–63 (1972).

Morrison, D.F.: Multivariate statistical methods (McGraw Hill, New York 1967).

Shagass, C.: Evoked brain potentials in psychiatry (Plenum Press, New York 1972).

Shagass, C.; Ornitz, E.M.; Sutton, S.; Tueting, P.: Event related potentials and psychopathology; in Callaway, Tueting, Koslow, Event-related brain potentials in man, pp. 443–496 (Academic Press, New York 1978a).

Shagass, C.; Roemer, R.A.; Straumanis, J.J.: Deviant topography of sensory evoked potentials in psychosis. Adv. biol. Psychiat., vol. 4, pp. 94–101 (Karger, Basel 1980a).
Shagass, C.; Roemer, R.A.; Straumanis, J.J.; Amadeo, M.: Evoked potential correlates of psychosis. Biol. Psychiat. *13:* 163–184 (1978b).
Shagass, C.; Roemer, R.A.; Straumanis, J.J.; Amadeo, M.: Spatial distribution of sensory evoked potentials in psychiatric disorders; Callaway, Lehmann, Human evoked potentials: Applications and problems, pp. 347–362 (Plenum Publishing Co., Ltd., New York 1979a).
Shagass, C.; Roemer, R.A.; Straumanis, J.J.; Amadeo, M.: Temporal variability of somatosensory, visual, and auditory evoked potentials in schizophrenia. Archs gen. Psychiat. *36:* 1341–1351 (1979b).
Shagass, C.; Roemer, R.A.; Straumanis, J.J.; Amadeo, M.: Topography of sensory evoked potentials in depressive disorders. Biol. Psychiat. *15:* 183–207 (1980b).
Shagass, C.; Schwartz, M.: Visual cerebral evoked response characteristics in a psychiatric population. Am. J. Psychiat. *121:* 979–987 (1965).
Shagass, C.; Straumanis, J.J.; Roemer, R.A.; Amadeo, M.: Evoked potentials of schizophrenics in several sensory modalities. Biol. Psychiat. *12:* 221–235 (1977).

Charles Shagass, MD, Eastern Pennsylvania Psychiatric Institute, Henry Avenue & Abbottsford Road, Philadelphia, PA 19129 (USA)

Adv. biol. Psychiat., vol. 9, pp. 50–56 (Karger, Basel 1982)

Visual Evoked Potential Topography in Patients with Schizophrenia and Normal Controls

M. S. Buchsbaum, A. C. King, J. Cappelletti, R. Coppola, D. P. van Kammen

Biological Psychiatry Branch (Chief: *W. E. Bunney, Jr.*), National Institute of Mental Health, Bethesda, Md., USA

Introduction

Smaller amplitude evoked potentials (EPs) have generally been found in patients with schizophrenia, whether visual, auditory or somatosensory EPs are studied [for review see *Buchsbaum,* 1977]. A recent large study using all three modalities confirmed this as well [*Shagass* et al., 1977]. This trend has been reported for most EP components and at various recording positions, making a specific neuropsychological deficit hard to establish. If all components are diminished in all areas, then some generalized increase in response latency variability at primary areas might be hypothesized which would reduce average EP amplitude diffusely over the cortex. However, in the only systematic analysis of full electrode arrays, *Shagass* et al. [1979] report topographic differences in EP variability between schizophrenics and normals. Visual EPs for schizophrenics did show significant left-sided topographic patterns with high variability in comparison with normals mainly in central and temporal leads for a 151–450 ms epoch. Thus, an evaluation of left hemisphere visual EP amplitude on a component-by-component basis would complement these variability studies.

Subjects and Methods

A sample of 6 patients (4 men and 2 women, ages 18–30) who were hospitalized as inpatients at the NIH Clinical Center participated in the study. All had been medication-free for at least 2 weeks, and 5 were right-handed. All patients were in good physical health and none had clinically significant abnormalities evident on physical examination or lab tests which

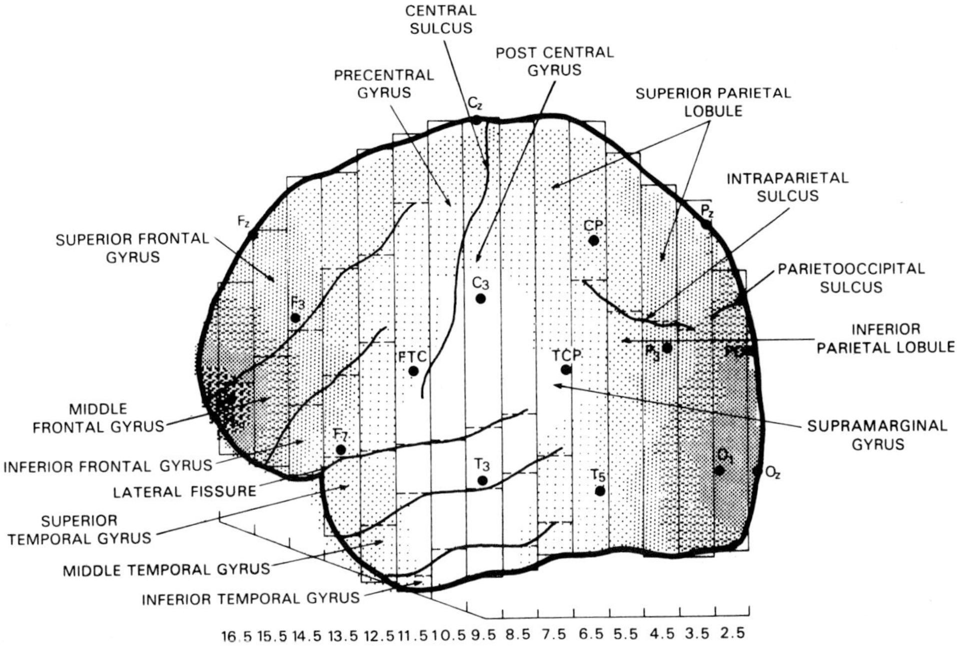

Fig. 1. Visual EP maps for N120 component for data from 7 normal volunteers. Projections of electrode positions developed from cross-sectional atlas.

included EEG, skull X-rays or CT head scan. Patients were diagnosed on the basis of both the Diagnostic and Statistical Manual of Mental Disorders [American Psychiatric Association, 1980] and Research Diagnostic Criteria (RDC) [*Spitzer* et al., 1978] by the patient's psychiatrist and diagnosis was confirmed by another staff psychiatrist.

13 normal volunteers approximately age- and sex-matched served as controls. The EP stimuli were four intensities of light flashes (2, 30, 80 and 240 ft La) and four intensities of tones each presented 64 times in a randomized sequence at 1-second intervals [*Buchsbaum* et al., 1981]. EEG was recorded from 16 channels all on the left side, including all 10–20 system locations, midline F_z-C_z-P_z-O_z and four additional electrode locations added to provide greater resolution of the posterior cortex. These are placed at the centers of squares formed by connecting P_3-P_2-O_z-O_1 (PO), C_3-C_z-P_z-P_3 (CP), T_3-C_3-P_3-T_5 (TCP), and F_7-F_3-C_3-T_3(FTC). For the cortical mapping experiments, EPs were first detrended using linear regression and then digitally filtered to remove frequencies below 4 Hz and above 30 Hz as described (with a different bandpass) elsewhere [*Lavine* et al., 1980]. Eye movements and artifacts were monitored using lead F_p1; trials exceeding a threshold were automatically excluded from the average for all leads. Individuals exceeding a 50 % trial loss on any condition were excluded. The 16 values were then used to interpolate values over the entire scalp area as described elsewhere [*Buchsbaum* et al., 1982]. EPs were measured as described elsewhere [*Buchsbaum*

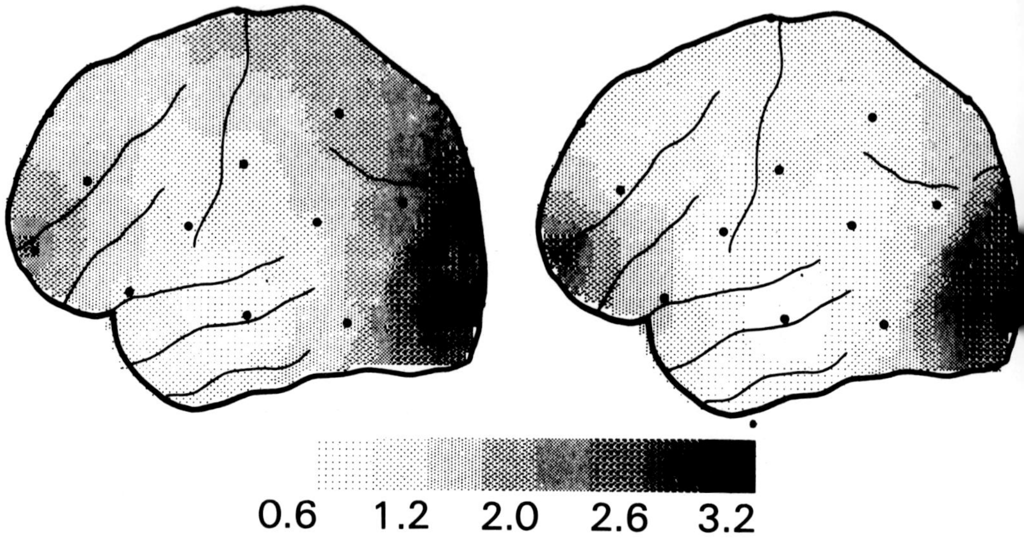

Fig. 2. P100 component in 13 normal controls *(a)* and 6 schizophrenics *(b)*. Gray scale shows amplitude in microvolts. Note similar distributions, but darker gray appearance of normal map.

et al., 1977]; by area integration for P100 (76–112 ms), N120 (116–152 ms) and P200 (168–240 ms). Figure 1 illustrates a typical topographic map with anatomical landmarks developed from a cross-sectional atlas study [*Buchsbaum* et al., 1982]. Average maps were calculated from amplitude averages for each of the 16 leads.

All subjects were required to count the number of visual stimuli which were of the same intensity ignoring intervening tones, as described elsewhere [*Schechter and Buchsbaum,* 1973]. Two other tasks were also done with the same stimulus sequence [*Buchsbaum* et al., 1981], but only the data from the light attention task will be reported here.

Results

As widely reported, smaller visual EP amplitudes were found in the schizophrenic patients for all three peaks. This amplitude reduction is apparent in figures 2–4 as a lighter density. For P100 and P200, topographic differences between patient groups seem less pronounced than amplitude differences, although P200 appears to extend further back into the parietal area. In contrast, the N120 difference in topography is more marked with schizophrenic/normal differences being primarily in temporal and parietal regions (fig. 5).

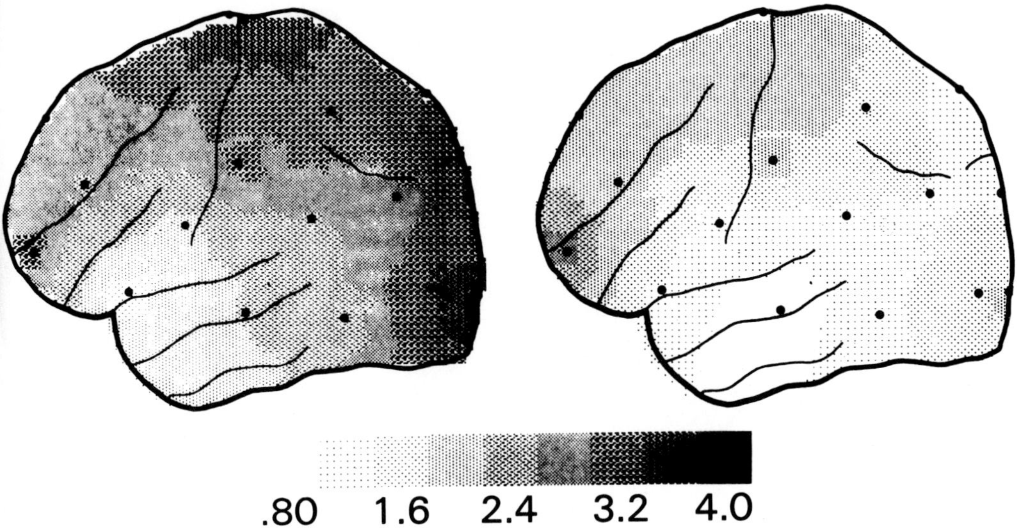

Fig. 3. N120 component distribution in the same individuals again shows all over darker (large amplitude) pattern of P100. However, N120 appears as a central-parietal-occipital band along the upper posterior edge in normals *(a)* whereas schizophrenics *(b)* show a gap in this region.

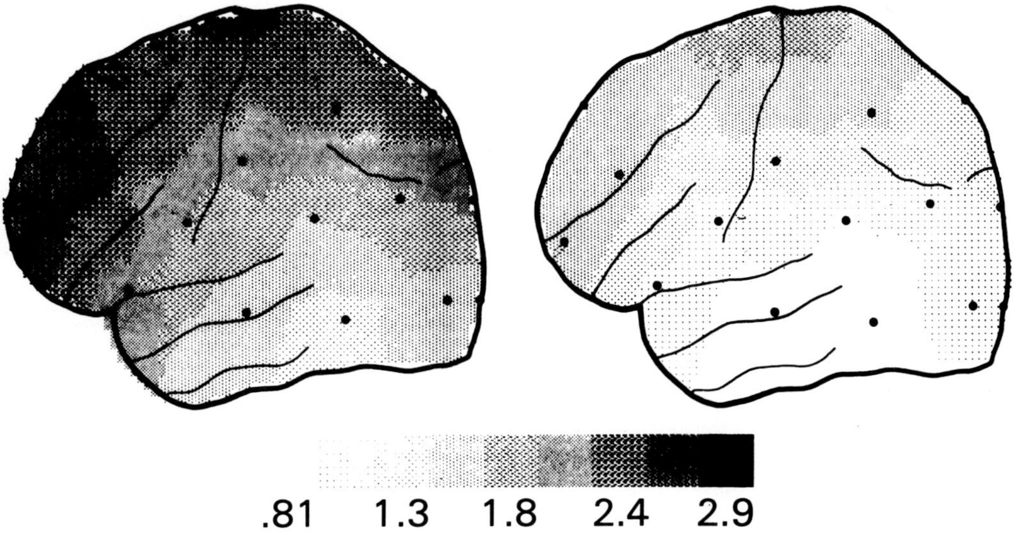

Fig. 4. P200 component distribution shows markedly smaller amplitudes (lighter values) in schizophrenics *(b),* although vertex maximum pattern is not dissimilar to normals *(a).*

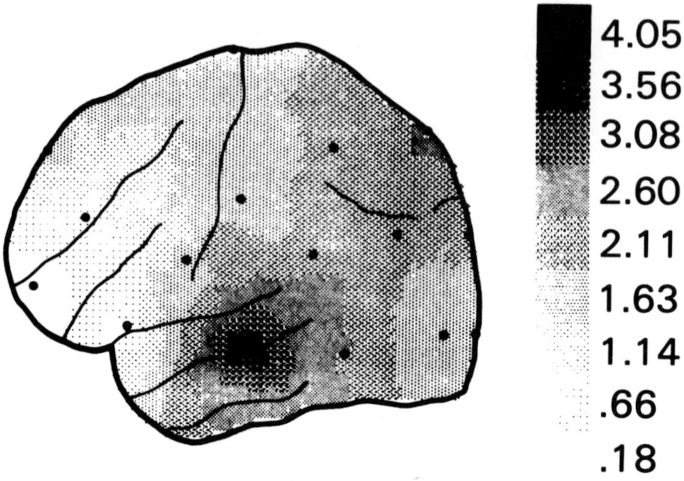

Fig. 5. t values from unpaired t tests on amplitudes of N120 component, intensity 1. t values were computed for each lead and then used for map interpolation. A temporal and parietal region of significance ($p < 0.05$, 2-tailed) is seen. Note absence of any frontal effect.

EP amplitude differences were confirmed by t tests on each component (3) lead (16) and intensity (4) for a total of 196 tests. Of these, 185 were in the predicted direction of normals > schizophrenics, 95 reaching statistical significance ($p < 0.05$, 1-tailed). Over all components intensity 1 reached significance the most often, and thus is shown in the figures. For intensity 1, leads P_z, P_3, and TCP reached statistical significance for P100, N120 and P200 ($p < 0.05$, unpaired t test). Significant amplitude differences at low (intensity 1), but not high (intensity 4) light levels were found for C_z, C_3, FTC and CP; such specific low intensity effects are commonly found with selective attention tasks. Patient/normal differences were not significant for F_p1 for any component (by t test), suggesting little if any contribution by eye movement artifacts.

Discussion

The results confirm the many existing studies of low EP amplitude in patients with schizophrenia with a suprisingly low sample size. Finding the largest number of significant t tests for P_z, P_3 and T_5, and the smallest for F_p1

mitigates against eye movement or blinks as sources of the effect, as does the shape of the t value distribution in figure 5.

Comparison of our data with the variability data of *Shagass* et al. [1979] shows similarity to their figure 7 where T_5 and T_3 also show the largest patient/normal differences in variability (they did not report P_3 or P_z). It may be that our P100 and P200 differences may reflect these areas having more variable and, therefore, lower amplitude average EPs.

It should be noted that *Shagass* et al. [1980] report no significant topographic differences in visual EP amplitude distribution (except for P300). Their use of checkerboard stimuli or the absence of a specific task could explain this difference. The N120 component with its topographic pattern differing between patients and normals seems to indicate a differing neurophysiological process, perhaps related to attentional processing. Pilot work indicated a specific parietal site for N120 enhancement with attention [*Buchsbaum* et al., 1981], and attentional mapping in a series of schizophrenic, is currently underway. We can at least recommend that visual EP studies of schizophrenia include T_5 or T_3 and P_z.

References

American Psychiatric Association. DSM-III: Diagnostic and Statistical Manual; 3rd ed. (APA, Washington 1980).

Buchsbaum, M. S.: The middle evoked response components and schizophrenia. Schizophr. Bull. *3:* 93–104 (1977).

Buchsbaum, M. S.; Coppola, R.; Gershon, E. S.; Kammen, D. P. van; Nurnberger, J. I.: Evoked potential measures of attention and psychopathology; in Perris, von Knorring, Advances in biological psychiatry, vol. 6 (Karger, Basel 1981).

Buchsbaum, M. S.; Post, R. M.; Bunney, W. E., Jr.: Average evoked responses in a rapidly cycling manic-depressive patient. Biol. Psychiat. *12:* 83–99 (1977).

Buchsbaum, M. S.; Rigal, F.; Coppola, R.; Cappelletti, J.; King, C.; Johnson, J.: A new system for gray-level surface distribution maps of electrical activity. Electroenceph. clin. Neurophysiol. *53:* 237–242 (1982).

Lavine, R. A.; Buchsbaum, M. S.; Schechter, G.: Human somatosensory evoked responses: effects of attention and distraction on early components. Physiol. Psychol. *8:* 405–408 (1980).

Schechter, G. A.; Buchsbaum, M. S.: The effects of attention, stimulus intensity and individual differences on the average evoked response. Psychophysiology *10:* 392–400 (1973).

Shagass, C.; Roemer, R. A.; Straumanis, J. J.: Amadeo, M.: Temporal variability of somatosensory, visual, and auditory evoked potentials in schizophrenia. Archs gen. Psychiat. *36:* 1341–1351 (1979).

Shagass, C.; Roemer, R.A.; Straumanis, J.J.: Deviant topography of sensory evoked potentials in psychosis; in Perris, von Knorring, Adv. biol. Psychiat., vol. 4, pp. 94–101 (Karger, Basel 1980).
Shagass, C.; Straumanis, J.J.; Roemer, R.A.; Amadeo, M.: Evoked potentials of schizophrenics in several sensory modalities. Biol. Psychiat. *12:* 221–235 (1977).
Spitzer, R.; Endicott, J.; Robins, E.: Research diagnostic criteria: rationale and reliability. Archs gen. Psychiat. *35:* 773–782 (1978).

M.S. Buchsbaum, MD, Room 2N-212, Clinical Center, National Institute of Mental Health, Bethesda, MD 20205 (USA)

Adv. biol. Psychiat., vol. 9, pp. 57–62 (Karger, Basel 1982)

A Critical Examination of Augmenting/Reducing Methodology in Schizophrenic Patients and Controls

J. F. Connolly[1], *J. H. Gruzelier*

Department of Psychiatry, Charing Cross Hospital Medical School, University of London, London, England

Introduction

Investigations of amplitude changes of the visual event-related potential (VEP) with flash intensity have shown that amplitudes do not increase monotonically with intensity in all subjects [1]. Subjects whose amplitudes increase have been termed 'augmenters' and those whose amplitudes decrease 'reducers' [2]. This typology has related to a plethora of issues. which we document elsewhere [1]. The present study was undertaken to clarify the following issues: (1) As so many techniques (e. g. time bands and linear slopes) have been used to define augmenting/reducing it was decided to test whether groups established by different methods were comparable. (2) Given the inverse relation between stimulus intensity and VEP latencies it was deemed advisable to determine if actual VEP peaks regularly occurred within the time bands assigned to them. Given the frequently-reported latency abnormalities in schizophrenics it was also thought important to ascertain if their VEP peaks were less likely to occur within appropriate time bands. (3) The entire VEP augmenting/reducing phenomenon and time band method are based on vertex recordings yet other sites have been used. As VEP characteristics vary topographically this experiment sought to determine whether the success of time bands also varied topographically.

[1] Wellcome Research Fellow

Methods and Subjects

The subjects were 22 healthy volunteers (11 men and 11 women) from the staff of Charing Cross Hospital and 16 unmedicated schizophrenics tested (11 men and 5 women). Groups were age-matched – the controls were 30.0 years and patients 31.2 years. All subjects were dextral [1] and had normal or corrected vision.

Six intensities of visual stimuli (flash: 20° horizontal × 16° vertical) were used: 0.31, 0.65, 1.25, 2.5 and 10 ft La as measured at the subject. Stimuli were presented in a Latin square design in blocks of 10 for each intensity. Stimulus duration was 500 ms and the interstimulus interval (ISI) was 500 ms. The interval between blocks of stimuli was variable between 5 and 15 s. The subject sat with eyes open and fixated on a point on a screen 122 cm away on which flashes were back-projected at eye level. The EEG (1–75) Hz half-amplitude band pass) was recorded with Ag/Ag Cl electrodes at Cz, 0_1, 0_2, T_3, T_4 with linked ears as reference. An electrode placed on the right arm served as ground. EOG was recorded throughout. 15 % of trials was the maximum for any subject lost due to EOG artefact. EOG artefacts did not correlate with stimulus intensity.

P100-N120 and N120-P200 peak-to-trough amplitudes were measured as well as the amplitude of each peak from a pre-stimulus baseline and its latency. In order to compensate for the shorter than usual time constant employed here time bands were adjusted by 8 ms. We found that the use of variable time constants did affect the success of the method which defines augmenting/reducing with set time bands [1], thought the general neglect of this issue [3, 4] might have suggested otherwise. Time bands were as follows: P100: 68–104; N120: 108–144; P200: 160–232.

In order to make direct comparisons with other work, P100 time band 'amplitudes' were obtained by calculating the mean voltage of the entire VEP epoch, subtracting the points within the time band from the mean voltage and calculating the mean of these deviations. Slopes were applied to the peak-to-trough values and to the P100 time band values. All slopes were calculated by the least squares method and a measure was obtained of the linearity of fit (the coefficient of determination). In those analyses involving slope measures subjects with positive slopes were classified as 'augmenters' and those with negative slopes as 'reducers'.

The method thought most appropriate to measure an augmenting or reducing stimulus intensity function was as follows. An augmenting pattern was defined as one which showed at vertex a monotonic increase in the P100-N120 peak-to-trough amplitude across the three highest intensities. The amplitude to the highest intensity was required to be the largest amplitude recorded. A reducing pattern was simply one which failed to meet the above criteria for augmenting.

Results

Time Bands an Slope Techniques

Table I presents the percentage of VEP peaks which occurred within the designated time band for each of the 5 electrode placements for both groups. While with few exceptions mean peak latencies to all intensities at all placements for the *grouped* data occurred within the specified time band

Table I. Percentages of VEP peaks occurring within specified time bands (see text for details)

Component	Group	T_3	T_4	C_z	O_1	O_2	
P100	patients	70	72	64	49	46	60.2
	controls	82	80	82	75	59	75.6
N120	patients	66	67	69	43	48	58.6
	controls	84	76	81	72	70	76.6
P200	patients	78	76	80	77	80	78.2
	controls	94	93	86	88	86	89.4

Schizophrenic patients 65.7; Normal controls 80.5

it is clear that: (1) the percentage of peaks occurring within the time bands is low; (2) percentages are lower for schizophrenic patients for P100 ($p<0.008$), N120 ($p<0.004$) and P200 ($p<0.004$); (3) there are large differences in percentages among the 5 placements; and (4) the percentages are lowest (especially for schizophrenics) for the peaks used to define augmenting/reducing (i.e. P100 and N120). In fact the percentage of peaks occurring within time bands was lower for schizophrenics than controls for each peak at every placement. Percentages also differed considerably between augmenters and reducers [data available from authors].

Should the time band continue to be used as an alternative to customary peak identification techniques it is important to establish if the methods produce similar results; an 85 % agreement might be considered acceptable. In the schizophrenic group 12.5 % of the sample had 85 % or more of their VEP peaks occur within the specified time bands. When the criterion was lowered to 75 % still only 31.3 % of the patients achieved this criterion. The corresponding values for controls are only 18 and 59 %. Thus, while time bands may appear acceptable for *grouped* data they clearly are inappropriate when used on individual subjects, the aim of the typology.

The next issue concerns an alternative approach, namely the validity of fitting a linear model to either peak-to-trough or time band amplitude

Table II. Agreement among methods of defining augmenters and reducers in patients and controls (in parentheses)

		A		
		augmenter	reducer	
B	augmenter	4 (1)	1 (2)	chi square = 3.2776, NS (0.0289, NS)
	reducer	2 (9)	9 (10)	percent agreement = 81 % (50 %)
		A		
		augmenter	reducer	
C	augmenter	2 (5)	0 (0)	chi square = 1.3714, NS (5.178, $p<0.05$)
	reducer	4 (5)	10 (12)	percent agreement = 75 % (77 %)
		B		
		augmenter	reducer	
C	augmenter	1 (1)	1 (4)	chi square = 0.0416, NS (0.0726, NS)
	reducer	4 (2)	10 (15)	percent agreement = 69 % (73 %)

Method A = P100–N120 slope; method B = P100 time band slope; method C = P100–N120 amplitude change.

changes across intensities. The mean coefficients of determination for values of patients and controls were low for the P100-N120 (0.33 and 0.30) and P100 time band (0.32 and 0.50) techniques indicating that the imposition of a linear function on amplitude changes across intensities is inappropriate. Thus, methods of defining a subject as an augmenter or reducer by amplitude-intensity slopes are invalid. The obvious next question is whether different methods of defining augmenting/reducing produce the same groups. Table II shows that whether a subject is labelled an augmenter or reducer varies with the method.

Discussion

The results raise several questions about the augmenting/reducing phenomenon as measured by evoked potentials. It has been shown, using the coefficient of determination, that the fitting of a straight line to VEP amplitude changes in individual subjects [2] is not a valid procedure. For this reason recent approaches which use this technique would have marginal relevance to earlier work not only due to differences in definitions (VEP vs. KFA) but also because of different methods of VEP assessment (amplitude changes vs. linear slopes) [1].

The validity of the time band method has also been questioned because the VEP peaks of individuals often occurred outside the group-derived time bands. This difficulty will also tend to vary with intensity and electrode placement; the latter problem is due to time bands being based on VEP peaks recorded at vertex. Thus, spurious data are inevitable when vertex-based time bands are used for VEPs recorded at other sites [5]. As hypothesised these effects were far more pronounced in the schizophrenic group.

Another problem with the time band methodology is baseline determination. The use of mean activity in the VEP epoch as the baseline is problematic. This type of baseline would be susceptible to producing artefactual results due to the occurrence of late VEP components (e.g. P300). It is rightly observed [4] that late components are unlikely in the augmenting/reducing paradigm. However, this may not address the real problem. *Any* peak which is affected by stimulus intensity and occurs later than the time band under study will influence such a baseline. A late negative VEP peak (latency 225–300 ms) has been shown to be sensitive to stimulus intensity [1]. Therefore, studies using an epoch baseline and measuring activity in P100, N140 and P200 time bands [5] are weakened inasmuch as the baseline will be affected by an unaccounted for peak. Similarly, experiments assessing just the P100 time band [3] are difficult to interpret as there are three intensity-sensitive peaks (N140, P200 and N225) affecting the epoch baseline. As a result P100 time band 'amplitude' changes are quite likely to be due to a shifting baseline attributable to one or several of these later peaks.

This experiment has demonstrated that there will be little correspondence in augmenter and reducer groups between studies utilising linear slopes [2] and those using time bands [3]. In fact, recent work [6] has shown that even when the same augmenter/reducer definition is used a subject's classification can change after nothing more than a short rest period. In conclusion, the time band method makes the following assumptions: (1) negligible topographic differences in peak latencies; (2) small between-subject latency differences; (3) negligible intensity-related changes in latencies; and (4) no intensity-related changes in peak amplitudes occurring after the time band under scrutiny. This experiment and others [1, 6] have demonstrated that none of these assumptions are valid.

References

1 Connolly, J.F.; Gruzelier, J.H.: Amplitude and latency changes in the visual evoked potential (VEP) to different stimulus intensities. Psychophysiology (to be published, 1982).

2 Buchsbaum, M.; Pfefferbaum, A.: Individual differences in stimulus intensity response. Psychophysiology *8:* 600–611 (1971).

3 Buchsbaum, M.S.; Haier, R.J.; Murphy, D.L.: Suicide attempts, platelet monoamine oxidase and the average evoked response. Acta psychiat. scand. *56:* 69–79 (1977).

4 Buchsbaum, M.; Coppola, R.: Signal-to-noise ratio and response variability in affective disorders and schizophrenia; in Begleiter, Evoked brain potentials and behavior, vol. 2 (Plenum Press, New York 1979).

5 Coursey, R.D.; Buchsbaum, M.; Frankel, B.L.: Personality measures and evoked responses in chronic insomniacs. J. abnorm. Psychol. *84:* 239–249 (1975).

6 Connolly, J.F.: The influence of passive and task conditions on intensity-related changes in exogenous visual event-related potentials (ERPs). Int. Symp. on the Psychological Significance of Event-Related Potentials, Zeist (1980).

Dr. J.F. Connolly, Department of Psychiatry, Charing Cross Hospital Medical School, Fulham Palace Road, London, W6 8RP (England)

Adv. biol. Psychiat., vol. 9, pp. 63–66 (Karger, Basel 1982)

Dose-Related Effects of Chlorpromazine on Psychometric and Electrophysiological Parameters in Wakefulness

J. M. Gaillard, S. Laurian, P. K. Le

Clinique Psychiatrique de l'Université de Lausanne, Hôpital de Cery, Prilly, Suisse

Introduction

Previous investigations have shown that chlorpromazine (CPZ) modifies paradoxical sleep (PS) differently as a function of the dose, in the rat and in man [*Kafi and Gaillard,* 1978; *Gaillard and Kafi,* 1979]. The production of this stage is facilitated by a low dose of the drug, and decreased by a higher dose. The facilitation of PS under a low dose of CPZ has been ascribed to preferential blockade of α_2-adrenoceptors, whereas the decrease observed under high dose probably reflects predominant blockade of α_1-adrenoceptors [*Kafi and Gaillard,* 1978]. A similar dose-response relationship has been detected in wakefulness: the completion of a logic test was faster under 25 mg of CPZ than under placebo, and slower under 75 mg [*Hartley and Couper-Smartt,* 1978]. Thus, the low dose acted as a stimulant rather than a sedative.

A number of experimental results indicate that brain catecholamine systems, particularly noradrenaline (NA), are involved in the regulation of PS and wakefulness [for review, see *Jouvet,* 1972]. Therefore, we investigated the effect of various doses of CPZ in normal subjects, by measuring a number of psychometric and electrophysiological parameters, in order to study the possible role of α_1- ad α_2-adrenoceptors in wakefulness.

Methods

10 paid male volunteers, 20–30 years old, were studied in the laboratory. After habituation to the recording procedure, 5 subjects (group I) received 0.5 and 1.5 mg/kg of CPZ in separate sessions, whereas the other 5 (group II) received 0.25 and 0.75 mg/kg.

Psychometric investigations before and 2 h after drug administration consisted of: (1) a 9-point scale of global feeling of tiredness and a 12-item index of alertness; (2) simple reaction time to random acoustic stimuli; (3) multiple-choice reaction time to acoustic and visual stimuli; the subject had to respond only to predetermined combinations; (4) the digit ordination test of Rey; the number of series of 7 random digits correctly ordinated was counted.

Spontaneous brain electrical activity (EEG) was recorded with eyes closed from four pairs of symmetrical electrodes (F3/F4, C3/C4, T3/T4 and O1/O2), referenced to the interconnected earlobe electrodes. After filtering (46 dB attenuation between 30 and 38 Hz), manual and automatic artifact rejection, the EEG was Fast Fourier transformed using a Med-80 computer. The signs of the difference between placebo and CPZ were computed for 64 EEG variables, including absolute and relative power in 4 spectral bands.

Evoked responses (ER) to flashes and checkerboard reversals were recorded from 7 unipolar derivations (F3/F4, C3/C4, CZ and O1/O2). ER sequences were filtered (30 Hz) and averaged after manual and automatic artifact rejection. Integrated amplitude and mean standard deviation over trials as a measure of variability were obtained for the average response to each type of stimulation. The signs of differences between placebo and CPZ were finally calculated for 28 ER variables.

A monophasic effect of CPZ was defined as a change of a given variable in the same direction under a low and high dose of CPZ, in at least 4 out of 5 subjects. Similarly, a biphasic effect was a change in the opposite direction under a low and high dose of the drug in at least 4 out of 5 subjects. For psychometric variables, the statistical estimation was realized using the unilateral sign test (S test) and the nonparametric Mann-Withney U test (U test).

Results

The index of alertness decreased, and the feeling of tiredness increased after the two large doses of 0.75 and 1.5 mg/kg (S test, $p<0.03$). These subjective parameters were not modified after the two small doses of CPZ compared to controls, but a significant change appeared in the comparison of pre- and postdrug differences of the two doses of 0.5 and 1.5 mg/kg (U test, $p<0.05$). Simple reaction time was significantly enhanced after only 0.75 mg/kg (S test, $p<0.03$), whereas no consistent effect was seen after the other doses. Again the comparison of 0.5 and 1.5 mg/kg revealed a significant difference (U test, $p<0.05$). The interindividual variability in complex reaction time and digit ordination was considerable, and prevented any significant modification to appear with respect to the control condition. However, in these two tests, the comparison of 0.5 and 1.5 mg/kg disclosed a significant effect of the dose (U test, $p<0.05$).

In group I, the most obvious change of spontaneous EEG under CPZ was an increase of the absolute value of theta activity in all derivations, an increase of delta in central regions and a decrease of beta in F4, C4 and T4.

Similar effects also appeared in group II, but in a smaller number of derivations. Thus, theta was increased in C4, O1 and O2, as was delta in C3, whereas beta was decreased in F3. Very few variations appeared in relative power densities. All these changes were monophasic, i.e. in the same direction under a low and high dose of CPZ.

However, in group I a few EEG parameters showed a biphasic effect as a function of the dose. The absolute value of alpha activity in C3, O1 and O2, and the absolute value of beta activity in O1 and O2 were enhanced under 0.5 and decreased under 1.5 mg/kg. Thus, in this group of subjects, 15 among the 64 EEG variables showed a monophasic effect, and 9 showed a biphasic effect. Among the set of 15 monophasic variables, 11 concerned theta and delta, but only one concerned alpha power. In contrast, among the 9 biphasic variables, only 2 concerned theta and delta, whereas 5 concerned alpha activity. In the second group of subjects receiving 0.25 and 0.75 mg/kg of CPZ, 9 variables were monophasic and only 1 was biphasic.

In group I a monophasic increase of variability of the ER to checkerboard reversals was consistently seen in 6 derivations under both doses of CPZ. However, the amplitude of the response to this type of stimulation was increased in O1 under 0.5 and decreased under 1.5 mg/kg of the drug, thus showing a biphasic effect. In group II, three variables were monophasic whereas none was biphasic.

Discussion

On the whole, the five psychometric tests indicated that a large dose of CPZ decreased subjective alertness, increased the feeling of tiredness, enhanced reaction time, and impaired the performance in digit ordination. However, the low dose of the drug did not induce any clear modification, a result which is not in favor of a biphasic effect. Interestingly, more consistent effects appeared in group I when the two doses of CPZ were compared than when each of them was compared to its corresponding control.

Obviously, CPZ induced more variations in spontaneous EEG than in ER. A rather clear difference appeared between slow activities of spontaneous EEG, which tended to increase after all doses of CPZ, and occipital alpha and beta activities which were enhanced under 0.5 mg/kg and decreased under 1.5 mg/kg with respect to the control condition. Thus, the power in these frequencies seems to be the only component of EEG to show a biphasic effect under CPZ.

However, it is known that a slight decrease of alertness may be accompanied by an increase of the abundance of alpha activity. When the level of alertness is further lowered, alpha activity decreases. Thus, a biphasic variation of this parameter may correspond to a monophasic change of alertness. The modification of beta activity as a function of alertness is less well understood.

The variability of ER was enhanced by CPZ in a monophasic way, whereas the amplitude of the responses to checkerboard reversals in the occipital area was greater under 0.5 and smaller under 1.5 mg/kg, compared to the control.

Taken together, these data indicate that most of the effect of CPZ in wakefulness is probably monophasic. It is not possible to rule out completely a biphasic effect on a few electrophysiological parameters, i. e. beta activity and amplitude of ER to checkerboard reversals. However, the evidence supporting such a view is much weaker than in sleep. It is possible that the larger individual variability in wakefulness, probably reflecting a larger number of different factors involved in the regulation of this state, makes impossible to see a biphasic effect as clearly as in sleep.

A monophasic effect of CPZ in wakefulness may indicate that the balance between α_1- and α_2-adrenoceptors is not the same as in sleep, and particularly in PS. Further experiments along this line may allow to define more precisely the role of α_2-adrenoceptors in wakefulness, a point of critical importance in the understanding of the regulation of alertness states.

References

Gaillard, J.-M.; Kafi, S.; Involvement of pre- and postsynaptic receptors in catecholaminergic control of paradoxical sleep in man. Eur. J. clin. Pharmacol. *15:* 83–89 (1979).

Hartley, L.; Couper-Smartt, J.: Paradoxical effects in sleep and performance of two doses of chlorpromazine. Psychopharmacology *58:* 201–205 (1978).

Jouvet, M.: The role of monoamines and acetylcholine-containing neurons in the sleep-waking cycle. Ergebn. Physiol. *64:* 166–307 (1972).

Kafi, S.; Gaillard, J.-M.: Biphasic effect of chlopromazine on rat paradoxical sleep: a study of dose-related mechanisms. Eur. J. Pharmacol. *49:* 251–257 (1978).

Dr. J.-M. Gaillard, Clinique Psychiatrique de l'Université de Lausanne, Hôpital de Cery, CH-1008 Prilly (Suisse)

Adv. biol. Psychiat., vol. 9, pp. 67–80 (Karger, Basel 1982)

The Acute Drug Effect as Predictor of Therapeutic Outcome: Neurophysiological/ Behavioral Correlations during Anxiolytic Therapy of Alcoholics

B. Saletu, J. Grünberger, M. Saletu, R. Mader, M. Karobath

Section of Pharmacopsychiatry (Head: Prof. *Bernd Saletu*), Psychiatric University Clinic of Vienna (Chairman: Prof. *P. Berner*), Vienna, Austria; Anton Proksch Institute (Prim. Dr. *R. Mader*), Vienna, Austria

Introduction

While it is generally acknowledged that changes in clinical symptomatology during pharmacotherapy of psychiatric patients are linked to changes in their brain activity which in turn are dependent on blood level alterations, there is a paucity of data supporting these assumptions. Correlations between drug-induced neurophysiological and behavioral changes could be demonstrated during neuroleptic treatment of chronic schizophrenic patients [*Saletu* et al., 1973 a, b; *Saletu*, 1976; *Itil* et al., 1975] and psychotic children [*Saletu* et al., 1975 a], further during amphetamine treatment of hyperkinetic children [*Saletu* et al., 1975 b] and during the therapy of chronic alcoholics with a new pyridodiazepine lopirazepam [*Saletu* et al., 1979]. The present double-blind study was carried out to investigate the clinical symptomatology, brain activity, psychometric performance and blood level of chronic alcoholics undergoing alcohol withdrawal before and during therapy with 2 pharmacokinetically different benzodiazepines (the short-acting lopirazepam and the long-acting prazepam) and to study specifically the relationship between changes in the aforementioned variables. Moreover, an attempt was made to replicate previous correlations suggesting that eventually it might be possible to predict a therapeutic outcome based on acute quantitative EEG and psychometric changes [*Saletu* et al., 1979].

Method

Population

42 male hospitalized patients with the diagnosis of alcohol dependency (ICD 303), in whom an anxiolytic drug therapy was indicated due to the expected withdrawal and anxiety syndrome, were included in the study after an informed consent was obtained. One more patient started the program but dropped out for nondrug-related reasons. At the onset of the double-blind study the patients had to be a minimum of 10 days off any psychoactive medication and at least 24 h off of alcohol. After the baseline investigation the patients were assigned randomly to anxiolytic drug therapy for 3 weeks with either lopirazepam or prazepam. They received in the neurophysiological laboratory one single oral dosage of 10 mg lopirazepam or 10 mg prazepam; thereafter the optimal daily dosage was titrated by the psychiatrist up to the end of the 1st week, while in the 2nd and 3rd week a maintenance dosage was administered according to a t.i.d. schedule. No other psychoactive drugs were allowed. Apart from the pharmacotherapy, the patients participated actively in psychotherapeutic (group therapy), sociotherapeutic and occupational therapy programs.

The mean age (± SD) of the lopirazepam group was 39.7 (8.1) years, and of the prazepam patients 36.6 (5.8) years; the average weight (± SD) was 71.05 (10.93) kg in the lopirazepam group and 74.81 (13.49) kg in the prazepam group; the mean height (± SD) of lopirazepam-treated patients was 172.3 (5.22) cm and of prazepam-treated patients 175.86 (6.47) cm.

In the 4th week the lopirazepam group (L) and the prazepam group (D = Demetrin®) was divided into 3 subgroups: 2 groups (with 7 patients each) were continued on active medication (LL and DD), 2 other groups (with 7 patients each) received placebo (LP and DP), while again 2 other groups (with 7 patients each) did not receive any drug (LO and DO). However, these data will be discussed elsewhere [*Saletu* et al., in press].

Blood Level Determination

10 mg venous blood samples were collected in heparinized plastic tubes before the morning medication (12 h after the last medication at 8 p.m.) on days 0, 7 and 21. The blood was centrifuged and the plasma frozen and kept at −20°C until analysis by a radioreceptor assay for benzodiazepines in plasma [*Skolnick* et al., 1979]. The latter technique permits the measurement of blood levels of receptor active compounds (drug and active metabolites). The obtained values were categorized within the following ranges: 1 = questionably positive (<30 ng/ml); 2 = lightly positive (31–100 ng/ml); 3 = positive (101–300 ng/ml); 4 = markedly positive (301–600 ng/ml); 5 = markedly positive (>600 ng/ml). Bilirubin, SGOT, SGPT, γ-GT and LDH were determined on days 0 and 21.

Clinical Evaluations

Clinical evaluations included the ECDEU Clinical Global Impression Rating Scale (CGI), the Hamilton Anxiety Rating Scale (HAM-A), the Zung Self-Rating Scale for Anxiety (SAS), the Zung Self-Rating Scale for Depression (SDS), the von Zerssen Befindlichkeits-skala for Self-Rating of Mood (Bf-S), the assessment of somatic findings and side effects as well as of weight, pulse, systolic and diastolic blood pressure and were carried out on days 0, 7 and 21 after the morning medication.

Psychometric Investigations

Psychometric investigations included the evaluation of attention [*Grünberger,* 1977]; psychomotor activity [*Grünberger,* 1977], and mood [*von Zerssen* et al., 1970] on days 1 and 21 (at the hours o and 2 after one single dosis) and on day 7; while the CFF, reaction time (ms) and the aftereffect (Archimedean spiral) were measured at the same times without day 7.

Neurophysiological Investigations

Neurophysiological investigations included a 5-min EEG before as well as 2 h after one oral single dose on days 1 and 21 [*Saletu* et al., in press]. The O2-Cz lead was analyzed off-line by a digital computer system (Intertechnique Plurimat S) utilizing power spectral density analysis programs. Following 38 EEG variables were calculated: absolute and relative power in 9 frequency bands, the combined δ and ϑ (DT), α (A) and β bands (B); total power; the dominant frequency in the α range in Hz, as well as the absolute (ABS) and relative power (REL); and finally the average frequency (AF) and frequency deviation (FD) in the δ and ϑ, α, β and total frequency range (T).

Statistical Analyses

Statistical analyses included the Anova, the Newman-Keuls test, t-test, the X^2 test, Friedman's rank Anova and the multiple Wilcoxon test, as well as regression and correlation analyses.

Results

Dosis and Blood Levels

The mean optimal daily doses ($\pm$ SD) at the end of the 1st week were 23.8 (10.7) mg in the lopirazepam group and 35 (18.2) mg in the prazepam group, while at the end of the 3rd week they were 22.6 (10.9) mg and 31.9 (11.5) mg, respectively. Thus, based on a milligram to milligram comparison, lopirazepam my be regarded as the slightly more CNS-active drug than prazepam. On the other hand, blood level analysis by a radioreceptor assay demonstrated that after 1 week of lopirazepam therapy blood levels slightly though significantly ($p < 0.01$, multiple Wilcoxon) increased, while surprisingly after 3 weeks neither a quantitatively nor statistically significant increase was found (table I). This stands in sharp contrast to prazepam which revealed a marked increase in blood levels in the 1st and 3rd weeks ($p < 0.01$, multiple Wilcoxon test).

Clinical Findings

Evaluation of the psychopathology based on the CGI, HAM-A, SAS, SDS demonstrated that the 2 treatment groups did not differ before the

Table I. Benzodiazepine blood levels, clinical symptomatology and psychometry before and during anxiolytic therapy of the alcohol withdrawal syndrome

	Lopirazepam (n = 21)				Prazepam (n = 21)				Inter-drug difference	
	0	2 h	7 days	21 days	0	2 h	7 days	21 days		
Blood level (score)	0.7		1.7••	0.9•	0.8		3.9••	3.9••	Δ 7^{++}	21^{++}
CGI (score)	4.9		3.6**	3.1**	4.9		3.7**	3.2**	n.s.	
HAM-A (score)	26.4		10.3**	5.8**	27.8		9.9**	8.1**	n.s.	
SAS (index)	54.8		38.6**	35.0**	53.3		38.6**	35.8**	n.s.	
SDS (index)	52.9		38.1**	36.2**	51.0		40.2**	36.6**	n.s.	
CFF, Hz	42.8	42.3		42.2	42.7	41.3*		41.9	n.s.	
After effect, s	9.3	8.7		8.2	9.4	7.6**		7.9**	n.s.	
Reaction time, ms	439	414		417*	461	440		399**	n.s.	
Attention (score)	429	383**	417	464	386	383	412	428*	Δ 2h^{+}	
Motor activity (score)	40.4	43.7	48.4**	50.7**	41.2	45.9	46.6	51.6**	n.s.	
Mood (Bf-S) (score)	25.8	18.9**	8.7**	7.3**	26.7	20.0**	9.9**	9.7**	n.s.	

Newman-Keuls: * $p < 0.05$; ** $p < 0.01$. Multiple Wilcoxon: • $p < 0.05$; •• $p < 0.01$. Wilcoxon: $^{++}$ $p < 0.01$. t test: $^{+}$ $p < 0.05$.

start of the therapy. After 1 week of lopirazepam or prazepam treatment, both patient populations exhibited a marked and highly statistically significant improvement in their symptomatology ($p < 0.01$, Newman-Keuls test), while further treatment until the end of the 3rd week resulted only in minimal additional improvement (table I). There were, however, no statistically significant differences between the two groups.

Evaluation of somatic findings, pulse rate, blood pressure and weight suggested that both compounds were very well tolerated. Laboratory findings including bilirubin, SGOT, SGPT, γ-GT and LDH showed in both treatment groups a marked and significant ($p < 0.05$-0.01, t-test) improvement after 3 weeks of therapy. This was seen both in terms of numbers of patients with abnormal values as well as in the actual change values of these variables [*Saletu* et al., in press]. Last but not least, one has to mention that even the abnormal values at the end of treatment period were mostly in the borderline range.

Psychometric Findings

Attention as measured by means of the total score of the AD test demonstrated a significant decrease 2 h after 1 single dosis of lopirazepam, while it improved at the end of the 3rd week increasing to scores above the baseline level (table I). The latter change was significant in the prazepam-treated group. There was a significant inter-group difference regarding the acute drug effect due to the different kinetics.

Psychomotor activity improved already slightly after the administration of one single dose of both compounds and markedly and significantly so at the end of the 1st and 3rd weeks of lopirazepam therapy and after 3 weeks of prazepam administration (table I).

Mood improved clinically and statistically already after 1 single dose and even further after chronic administration of both compounds (table I).

Critical flicker frequency (CFF) showed no changes in the lopirazepam group, while a slight decrease after 1 single dose but not after chronic administration of prazepam was noted (table I).

Aftereffect according to the Archimedean spiral tended to decrease after lopirazepam and significantly so after acute and chronic administration of prazepam indicating desactivation (table I).

Reaction time tended to improve already after 1 single dose of both compounds and was significantly shortened after 3 weeks treatment (table I).

Neurophysiological Findings

2 h after 1 single dose of *10 mg lopirazepam,* a marked and statistically significant ($p < 0.01$–0.05, Newman-Keuls test) increase in absolute and relative power of the β activity as well as an increase of average frequency was noted, while δ and ϑ activity tended to decrease (fig. 1).

2 h after *10 mg prazepam* the same type of changes were observed, but the latter did not reach the level of statistical significance (fig. 1). A comparison between the drug-induced changes revealed that the increase in absolute power of the β activities was significantly greater after 10 mg lopirazepam than after 10 mg prazepam, which is obviously due to the different pharmacokinetics of the 2 compounds.

After *3 weeks therapy with lopirazepam* the δ and ϑ decrease reached the level of statistical significance as did the α augmentation (fig. 1). As will be discussed, the α augmentation together with the increase of relative and absolute power in the α dominant frequency as well as the lack of a significant β increase came as a surprise for a benzodiazepine administered chronically over 3 weeks. Further significant changes were the increase in average frequency of β activities and the increase in the average frequency and decrease in the frequency deviation of the total activity.

After *3 weeks prazepam therapy,* the outstanding feature was the marked and highly significant increase in β activity both in terms of absolute and relative power (fig. 1). There was further a decrease of slow activity, increase of average frequency, decrease in frequency deviation of the total β activity and a trend towards a decrease of α activity as well as of relative and absolute power of the α dominant frequency. Thus, the two active compounds differed significantly in respect to their changes in α and β activity, relative and absolute power of the α dominant frequency, as well as in average frequency and frequency deviation.

Administration of *one additional superimposed single dosis of 10 mg lopirazepam* on the top of chronic administration results again in a marked increase of β activity, average frequency and frequency deviation in both the total activity and β activity, while α activity decreased (fig. 1). While these changes reached the level of statistical significance after lopirazepam as compared with the day 21, this is not the case after prazepam. Thus, the 2 drugs differed in several variables, such as slow α activity, β activity, average frequency and frequency deviation of β activity and the frequency deviation of total activity.

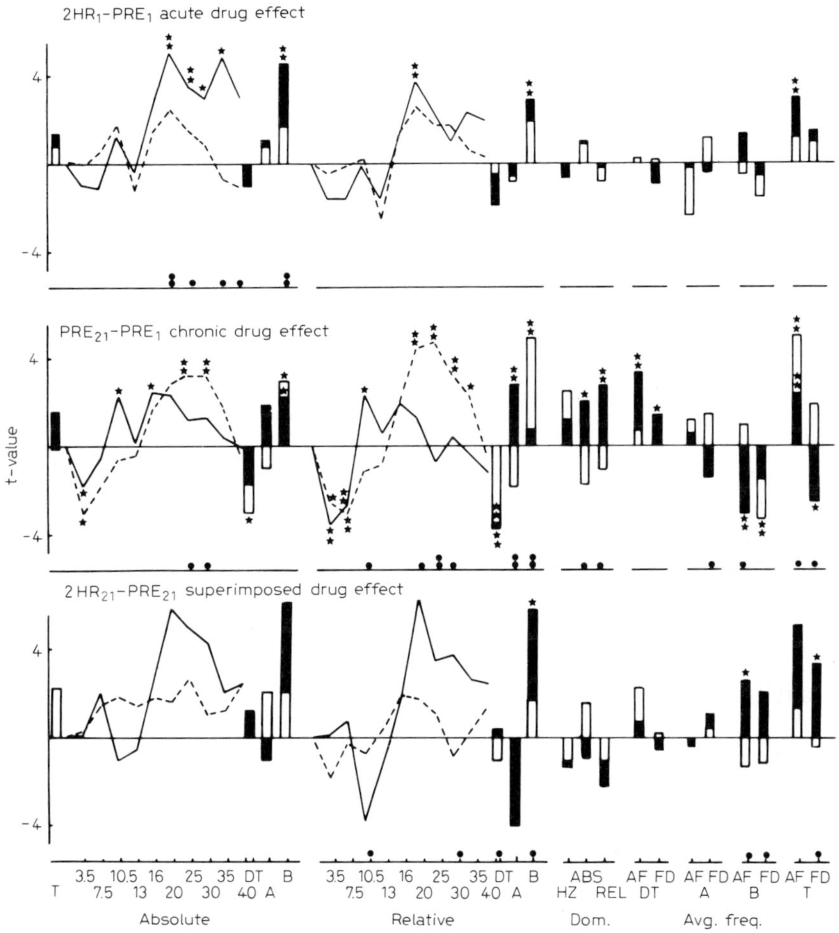

Fig. 1. Spectral analyzed EEG changes after acute and chronic anxiolytic therapy in the alcohol withdrawal syndrome (Cz-O2). 38 spectral analyzed EEG variables are shown in the abscissa, drug-induced changes as expressed in terms of t values are indicated in the ordinate. Changes from the pretreatment period are calculated by means of the Newman-Keuls test, inter-drug differences by the t test. Solid lines represent the lopirazepam group, interrupted lines the prazepam group. Newman-Keuls: * $p<0.05$; ** $p<0.01$; t test: • $p<0.05$; •• $p<0.01$.

Table II. Correlations between blood level, clinical, EEG and psychometric changes after 3 weeks anxiolytic therapy of alcoholics (n = 42)

	EEG changes							blood	Psychometric changes					
	TP	β_2	$\delta + \vartheta$	α	β	AF	FD	level	AD	FM	Bf	SP	CFF	RT
Clinical														
CGI	−0.27*		0.27*						−0.38**			0.39**	−0.30*	0.25
SDS		0.34*											−0.30*	
HAM-A		0.27							−0.30*	−0.35**				
SAS									−0.27*	−0.34*				
Blood level	−0.35*	0.24		−0.41**	0.46**	0.42**	0.42**			0.25				
Psychometric														
AD (attention)			−0.29*	0.29*										
FM (motor activity)									0.40**					
Bf (mood)														
SP (arch. spiral)	−0.26*						0.28*				0.25			
CFF														
RT (reaction time)														

* $p < 0.05$; ** $p < 0.01$.

Behavioral-Neurophysiological Correlations during Therapy

Regression and correlation analysis between changes in blood levels, clinical, psychometric and quantitative EEG variables after 3 weeks of treatment demonstrated a significant relationship between pharmacokinetics and pharmacodynamics as well as between alterations in brain activity and behavior. Of the 7 quantitative EEG variables selected for correlation analysis (total power = TP; relative power in 16–20 cps activity = β_2; combined δ and ϑ band, α band and β band; average frequency = AF and frequency deviation = FD), 5 were significantly and 1 borderline correlated to plasma levels (table II). The higher the plasma levels, the smaller the amplitude increase, the greater the increase in β activity, average frequency and frequency deviation and the more decrease in α activity in the EEG as well as the better the psychomotor performance in psychometry. There were few correlations between clinical changes and EEG alterations: the more decrease in δ and ϑ activity and the more increase in total power, the better the clinical improvement in the global score. The less β increase, the more decrease in HAM-A and SDS scores. On the other hand, there were more correlations between clinical and psychometric variables: the better the clinical improvement as reflected in the CGI, HAM-A, SAS and SDS scores, the better the attention, motor activity, reaction time and the higher the CFF. Significant neurophysiological-psychometric correlations were: the less slow and the more α activity, the better the attention; the greater the average frequency and the less amplitude increase, the longer the aftereffect (Archimedean spiral) suggesting CNS activation. Finally, there were also significant correlations between psychometric variables: the better the attention, the better the psychomotor performance; the lower the Befindlichkeits score, the less activated were the alcoholic patients after 3 weeks of therapy.

Acute Drug Effect as Predictor of Therapeutic Outcome

Correlating the acute changes in EEG and psychometric variables after single doses of 10 mg lopirazepam or prazepam with clinical changes after 3 weeks of chronic treatment, we found the following significant relationships: the more β increase, α decrease and increase in average frequency after single doses in EEG, the better the therapeutic outcome as seen by the decrease in Hamilton or Zung anxiety score after 3 weeks of treatment (table III). Similarly, the more improvement one gets with one single dose in attention and psychomotor activity, the better the results in the Zung depression and Hamilton anxiety ratings after chronic treatment. A

Table III. Acute EEG and pychometric drug effects as predictors of therapeutic outcome in alcoholics (n = 42)

Chronic change (after 3 weeks)	Acute change (after 2 h)											
	EEG						psychometric					
	TP	β_2	$\delta + \vartheta$	α	β	AF	AD	FM	Bf	SP	CFF	RT
Clinical												
CGI 7												
CGI 21										0.33*	−0.41**	0.30*
SDS 7							−0.33*					
SDS 21							−0.50**				−0.40**	
HAM-A 7												−0.28*
HAM-A 21		−0.26*						−0.26*			−0.31*	
SAS 7		−0.35*		0.26*								
SAS 21		−0.38**		0.26*	−0.38**	−0.29*						
Psychometric												
AD 7 (attention)							0.33*					
AD 21							0.37**					
FM 7 (motor activity)								0.34*				
FM 21												
Bf 7 (mood)	0.26*		−0.28*	0.27*					0.50**			
Bf 21			−0.38**	0.27*					0.42**			
SP 21 (arch. spiral)	−0.34*			−0.36						0.73**		
CFF 21								0.30	0.47**		0.70**	
RT 21 (reaction time)												0.57**

* p <0.05; ** p <0.01.

decrease in α activity as well as an increase in slow activities was associated with an improvement in mood after 3 weeks of therapy. The less amplitude increase, the better the mood score and aftereffect after long-term treatment.

The highest correlations, however, were seen within one specific group of variables – the psychometric variables (table III).

Discussion

Our psychiatric and psychometric investigations demonstrated that the psychopathology and performance of alcohol-addicted patients undergoing alcohol withdrawal improved markedly and significantly during 3-week treatment with two anxiolytics – lopirazepam and prazepam. While certainly a spontaneous decline of symptomatology has to be considered in abstinent alcoholics especially in the 3rd week of therapy (and even more so as they participated also in psychotherapeutic, sociotherapeutic and occupational therapeutic programs), the improvement within the 1st week seems to be drug-related, as during this period of alcohol withdrawal a deterioration of clinical symptomatology in the untreated patients usually occurs [*Schuckit,* 1979]. Thus, in our present double-blind (phase 2) study we could replicate data of the preceding (phase 1) open study demonstrating a reduction in anxiety of about 62 % on day 2 of lopirazepam treatment, while at the end of the 1st week treatment the percentage increased to 71 % [*Saletu* et al., 1979]. It further confirms even earlier statements by us based on pharmaco-EEG and psychometric studies in normals [*Grünberger and Saletu,* 1978; *Saletu* et al., 1980] that lopirazepam is (1) CNS active as compared with placebo; (2) is a tranquilizer; (3) acts shortly in doses of 3, 5 and 10 mg up to the 4th, 6th and 8th hour, and is (4) slightly more effective than prazepam on a milligram to milligram basis, although one has to consider the different pharmacokinetics. Indeed, in the present study titration of the optimal dosage supports our pharmaco-EEG predictions.

Our findings concerning the lack of benzodiazepine-receptor binding activity 12 h after the last dosage of lopirazepam even after chronic administration over 3 weeks suggests that lopirazepam is indeed a rapidly acting benzodiazepine with a short invasion and a rapid elimination as opposed to the long-acting prazepam. This was also substantiated by our quantitative EEG data, as lopirazepam failed to induce the β augmentation and α attenuation known as typical for anxiolytics [*Fink,* 1975; *Saletu,* 1976] even after 3 weeks of chronic administration (although 12 h after the last dosage), while these characteristic alterations were clearly present when the recordings were obtained 2 h after single doses.

Regression and correlation analysis demonstrated that EEG changes were closely linked to changes in blood levels: the higher the plasma levels, the more β activity, the higher the average frequency, the less α activity and the smaller the amplitudes in the EEG. This confirm impressively earlier EEG and blood level correlations obtained by us with another benzodiazepine oxazepam [*Saletu and Grünberger,* 1979] as well as those of *Fink* [1975] after diazepam and bromazepam. Correlations between clinical and neurophysiological data were less impressive, while there were no correlations between blood levels and clinical/psychometric changes. This might be at least partly due to the fact that blood sampling and EEG recordings were done before the administration of the morning dosage, while clinical evaluation was carried out thereafter. That psychometric and clinical data correlate well comes as no surprise as psychometric tests concentrate on specific aspects of the total clinical syndrome.

Most interestingly seems to us the fact that we could confirm an earlier hypothesis about the prognostic value of the quantitative pharmaco-EEG regarding therapeutic outcome [*Saletu* et al., 1979]. In this past study we had observed: the greater the increase in average frequency 2 h after administration of one single oral dosis of 10 mg lopirazepam, the more pronounced the clinical improvement (Zung SAS score) in alcoholic patients after 3 weeks of chronic therapy. This correlation could be replicated in the present study even in the same variables, while additional predictors were identified in other neurophysiological and psychometric variables. Thus, the more sensitive a patient reacts to a single dosis of a certain compound, the better are his chances for clinical improvement with long-term treatment.

Summary

The psychopathology, psychometric performance and brain activity of 42 chronic alcoholics undergoing alcohol withdrawal were investigated before and during a 3-week treatment with 2 pharmacokinetically different benzodiazepines – the short-acting lopirazepam and the long-acting prazepam. A marked and highly significant improvement in psychopathology and psychometric performance as well as good drug tolerance was noted already at the end of the 1st week, while thereafter only a slight additional improvement was observed. Blood level investigations by a radioreceptor assay demonstrated that even after a 3-

week treatment with lopirazepam, blood levels obtained in the morning (12 h after the evening medication) were very low, while plasma levels of the long-acting prazepam remained high. This pharmacokinetic difference was also reflected in the spectral-analyzed EEG as in the acute drug trials only lopirazepam exhibited a typical anxiolytic profile, while after chronic administration the results were just the opposite. Regression and correlation analyses demonstrated that neurophysiological changes were closely linked to blood level alterations, while this was not the case with clinical changes. Finally, it was found that acute neurophysiological and psychometric changes after single dose administration could eventually serve as prognostic indicators for therapeutic outcome.

References

Fink, M.: Cerebral electrometry-quantitative EEG applied to human pharmacology; in Dolce, Künkel, Computerized EEG analysis, pp. 271–288 (Fischer, Stuttgart 1975).

Grünberger, J.: Psychodiagnostik des Alkoholkranken. Methodischer Beitrag zur Bestimmung der Organizität in der Psychiatrie (Maudrich, Wien 1977).

Grünberger, J.; Saletu, B.: Zur Anwendung des quantitativen Pharmako-EEG und der Psychometrie in der Klinischen Psychopharmakologie; in Erzigkeit, Lehrl, Blaha, Heerklotz, Messung und Messverfahren in der Psychopathologie, pp. 373–380 (Vless, Vaterstetten-München 1978).

Itil, T. M.; Marasa, J.; Saletu, B.; Davis, S.: Computerized EEG: predictor of outcome in schizophrenia. J. nerv. ment. Dis. *160:* 188–203 (1975).

Saletu, B.; Psychopharmaka, Gehirntätigkeit und Schlaf (Karger, Basel 1976).

Saletu, B.; Grünberger, J.: Evaluation of pharmacodymanic properties of psychotropic drugs: quantitative EEG, psychometric and blood level investigations in normals and patients. Pharmacopsychiatry *12:* 45–58 (1979).

Saletu, B.; Grünberger, J.; Linzmayer, L.; Stadler, R.: Classification and assessment of cerebral bioavailability of lopirazepam (D-12524) by quantitative EEG and psychometric analysis. Arzneimittel-Forsch. *30:* 513–518 (1980.

Saletu, B.; Itil, T. M.; Arat, M.; Akpinar, S.: Long-term clinical and quantitative EEG effects of clopenthixol in schizophrenics: clinical-neurophysiological correlations. Int. Pharmacopsychiat. *8:* 193–207 (1973 a).

Saletu, B.; Saletu, M.; Grünberger, J.; Mader, R.: Drawing inferences about the therapeutic efficacy of drugs in patients from their CNS effect in normals: comparative quantitative pharmaco-EEG and clinical investigations; in Saletu, Berner, Hollister, Neuropsychopharmacology, pp. 393–407 (Pergamon Press, Oxford 1979).

Saletu, B.; Saletu, M.; Itil, T. M.: The relationships between psychopathology and evoked responses before, during and after psychotropic drug treatment. Biol. Psychiat. *6:* 45–74 (1973 b).

Saletu, B.; Saletu, M.; Simeon, J.; Marasa, J.: Fluphenazine treatment in the psychotic child: clinical-evoked potential correlations. Compreh. Psychiat. *16:* 265–278 (1975 a).

Saletu, B.; Saletu, M.; Simeon, J.; Viamontes, G.; Itil, T. M.: Comparative symptomatological nd evoked potential studies with *d*-amphetamine, thioridazine and placebo in hyperkinetic children. Biol. Psychiat. *10:* 253–275 (1975 b).

Saletu, M.; Saletu, B.; Grünberger, J.; Mader, R.; Karobath, M.: Clinical symptomatology and computerized analyzed EEG before, during and after anxiolytic therapy of alcohol withdrawal patients. Int. Pharmacopsychiat. (in press, 1982).

Schuckit, M. A.: Drug and alcohol abuse (Plenum Press, New York 1979).

Skolnick, P.; Goodwin, F. K.; Paul, S. N.: A rapid and sensitive radioreceptor assay for benzodiazepine in plasma. Archs gen. Psychiat. *36:* 78–80 (1979).

Zerssen, V. D. von; Koeller, D. M.; Rey, E. R.: Die Befindlichkeitsskala (BF-S) – ein einfaches Instrument zur Objektivierung von Befindlichkeitsstörungen, insbesondere im Rahmen von Längsschnittuntersuchungen. Arzneimittel-Forsch. *20:* 915–918 (1970).

Univ. Prof. Dr. Bernd Saletu, Head, Psychiatrische Universitätsklinik, Währingergürtel 74–76, A-1090 Vienna (Austria)

Adv. biol. Psychiat., vol. 9. pp. 81–86 (Karger, Basel 1982)

Effect of Imipramine and Zimelidine on the Augmenting-Reducing Response of Visual-Evoked Potentials in Healthy Volunteers[1]

L. von Knorring

Department of Psychiatry, Umeå University, Umeå, Sweden

In an early study by *Redmond* et al. [1975] in which monkeys were used, it was shown that changes in visual-evoked potentials (VEP) could be produced by the administration of substances influencing the turnover of the biogenic amines. Later, *Gottfries* et al. [1976] found that psychiatric patients with low concentrations of 5-HIAA in CFS had a more pronounced augmenting response in VEP than patients with high concentrations of 5-HIAA. The results were confirmed in later studies [*von Knorring* et al., 1980; *von Knorring and Perris,* 1981]. Furthermore, in a double-blind, placebo-controlled trial in chronic pain patients, it was shown that zimelidine, a rather specific serotonin reuptake inhibitor, changed the augmenting-reducing response of VEP in the direction of reduction [*von Knorring* et al., 1980]. Thus, it seems as if the augmenting-reducing response in VEP is related to changes in the serotoninergic pathways, while no relationship has been found with the noradrenaline metabolite, MOPEG, in CFS [*von Knorring and Perris,* 1981]. Thus the aim of the present study has been to evaluate the effect of produced changes in the noradrenergic and the serotoninergic systems on the augmenting-reducing response of different components in VEP.

[1] Supported in part by grants from the Swedish Medical Research Council (grants No. 2568, 5740) and by a grant from Astra Pharmaceuticals, Sweden.

Material and Methods

Subjects. 20 healthy volunteers, 8 male and 12 female, with a mean age of 30.9 years (age range 20–41 years) participated in the study.

Plan of the Investigation. The trial was performed as a double-blind, controlled randomized, cross-over study. The experimental investigations were performed at 10 a.m. on days 0, 2, 11, 20 and 28. The drugs were given at fixed times, 8 a.m., noon, 6 p.m.,on days 1–2, 10–11 and 19–20.

Drugs. Zimelidine was given in two different doses. However, in the present study, the interest is focused on the equipotent doses of imipramine (25 mg × 3 + 25 mg) and zimelidine (50 mg × 2 + 50 mg) [*Coppen* et al., 1979].

Accommodation Width and Saliva Secretion Rate. The accommodation width was determined by measuring the near point at emmetropi by means of a Jaeger IV text. The saliva secretion rate from both parotid glands was determined at rest and during stimulation [*von Knorring,* 1981].

Dryness in the Mouth. The subjective feeling of dryness in the mouth was assessed by means of a visual analogue scale [*von Knorring,* 1981].

Saliva Composition. In 10 of the subjects, the saliva composition, i. e. the relative content of electrolytes, proteins and glycoproteins was determined [*von Knorring and Mörnstad,* 1981].

Visual-Evoked Potentials. The subjects were presented visual stimuli of three intensities, 0.1, 0.2 and 0.6 J. The VEP were derived from a pair of electrodes applied over the occipital part of the dominant hemisphere (01; P3). After visual inspection, the positive peaks at about 100 and 200 ms and the negative peak at about 140 ms were identified and the peak to baseline amplitude determined in relation to the calibration signal. The methodology has been described earlier [*von Knorring* et al., 1980].

Statistics. The changes in saliva composition were corrected for changes in the saliva secretion rate. The coefficients used are described in detail elsewhere [*von Knorring and Mörnstad,* 1981]. Changes from baseline and differences between drugs were tested by means of t test of the difference.

Table I. Changes in accommodation width, self-rating of dryness in the mouth (visual analogue scale), saliva secretion rate at rest and saliva composition during short-term administration of imipramine 75 mg/day and zimelidine 100 mg/day: healthy volunteers, n = 20 (± SE)

	Baseline	Imipramine	Zimelidine
a Accommodation width, dryness in the mouth and saliva secretion			
Accommodation width, nearpoint in cm	12.5 ± 1.2	14.1 ± 1.3**	13.7 ± 1.4*
Dryness in the mouth, mm on a analogue scale	6.1 ± 2.3	34.8 ± 6.5***	24.5 ± 6.1*
Secretion rate at rest, ml/min	0.09 ± 0.02	0.02 ± 0.04***	0.06 ± 0.02
b Saliva composition			
Buffer capacity		+ 1.1 ± 0.6*	+ 0.7 ± 0.4
Electrolytes			
Na*		− 3.8 ± 5.5	− 3.9 ± 4.7
K*		+ 0.5 ± 0.9	+ 1.1 ± 0.8
Ca**		0.0 ± 0.0	0.0 ± 0.0
Protein		+ 20.0 ± 12.3	− 1.0 ± 9.4
Glycoproteins			
Sialic acid		+ 3.1 ± 1.1*	− 0.2 ± 0.7
Fucose		+ 16.3 ± 6.7	+ 8.5 ± 6.9
Hexoses		+ 19.3 ± 6.8*	+ 5.4 ± 5.9

* $p < 0.05$; ** $p < 0.01$; *** $p < 0.001$

Results

Both imipramine and zimelidine increased the nearpoint significantly, most pronounced for imipramine (table Ia). Both imipramine and zimelidine produced a significant increase in the subjective feeling of dryness in the mouth, most pronounced for imipramine (table Ia). Both imipramine and zimelidine decreased the saliva secretion rate at rest. However, the decrease was significant only for imipramine (table Ia). Imipramine, but not zimelidine in the corresponding dose, increased the buffer capacity significantly, increased the relative content of protein and glycoproteins. No changes were seen in the relative content of electrolytes (table Ib). At stimulus intensity 0.1 J no significant changes occurred in the latencies or the amplitudes of the components P_{100}, N_{140} or P_{200} of the VEP, neither for imipramine nor for zimelidine (table IIa, b). Zimelidine, but not imipramine, reduced the amplitude-intensity slope of the P_{100}–N_{140} component significantly. The effect seems to be in the N_{140} component, while no

Table II. Changes in amplitudes, latencies and amplitude-intensity slopes of VEP during short-term administration of imipramine 75 mg/day and zimelidine 100 mg/day: healthy volunteers, n = 20 (± SE)

	Baseline	Imipramine	Zimelidine
a Latencies			
Latency P_{100}	89.3 ± 2.7	90.8 ± 2.5	86.9 ± 2.4
Latency N_{140}	142.2 ± 3.9	138.9 ± 3.7	141.8 ± 3.6
Latency P_{200}	200.4 ± 4.4	200.3 ± 5.1	199.5 ± 4.6
b Amplitudes			
Amplitude P_{100}	6.2 ± 0.6	6.0 ± 0.7	6.7 ± 0.9
Amplitude N_{140}	2.7 ± 0.4	3.2 ± 0.5	3.4 ± 0.6
Amplitude P_{200}	1.3 ± 0.4	1.4 ± 0.5	1.7 ± 0.5
c Amplitude-intensity slopes			
P_{100}	+ 0.9 ± 1.2	− 0.4 ± 1.8	+ 0.1 ± 1.3
N_{140}	+ 2.2 ± 0.9	+ 2.6 ± 1.5	− 0.6 ± 0.8 *
P_{200}	+ 1.1 ± 0.7	+ 0.3 ± 0.6	+ 0.6 ± 0.7
P_{100}–N_{140}	+ 3.3 ± 1.4	+ 2.1 ± 2.0	− 0.5 ± 1.5 *

* $p < 0.05$

significant changes occurred in the amplitude-intensity slope of P_{100} component separately (table IIc). No significant changes occurred in the amplitude-intensity slope of the P_{200} component (table IIc).

Discussion

Imipramine is known to influence both the serotoninergic and the noradrenergic systems and to have a pronounced anticholinergic effect. Zimelidine is a rather specific serotonin reuptake inhibitor [*Siwers* et al., 1977] and has a less pronounced anticholinergic effect.

The results indicate that imipramine in the dose tested has a much more pronounced effect on accommodation width, subjective experience of dryness in the mouth and saliva secretion rate at rest than zimelidine in the corresponding dose. Thus, imipramine seems to have a much more pronounced effect on the cholinergic systems than zimelidine.

Imipramine also has a more pronounced effect on the saliva composition than zimelidine. The increase in protein and glycoproteins seems to be a result of an adrenergic stimulation and thus imipramine in the dose tested seems to have a much more pronounced effect on the adrenergic pathways than zimelidine in the corresponding dose. Thus, if imipramine had a more pronounced effect on the evoked potentials than zimelidine, the effect could be due to changes in the cholinergic or the adrenergic pathways, but if the most pronounced effect was produced by zimelidine, the effect would be due to changes in the serotoninergic pathways.

In the present study zimelidine, but not imipramine, significantly reduced the amplitude-intensity slope of the N_{140} component, also measurable as a significant reduction of the amplitude-intensity slope of the P_{100}–N_{140} component. Thus, the results are in line with earlier results indicating a reduction in the amplitude-intensity slope of the maximum amplitude of the VEP after zimelidine treatment [*von Knorring* et al., 1980]. The results also indicate that the amplitude-intensity slope is a more sensitive measure of changes in the serotoninergic systems than the amplitudes or latencies measured at a single stimulus intensity.

Summary

Imipramine (75 mg/day) and zimelidine (100 mg/day) were compared during short-term administration in a double-blind, controlled, cross-over trial in 20 healthy volunteers. Imipramine had the most pronounced effect on accommodation width and saliva secretion rate at rest, indicating a more pronounced anticholinergic effect than that of zimelidine. Imipramine, but not zimelidine in the corresponding dose, increased the relative content of protein and glycoproteins in the salive, indicating a more pronounced adrenergic effect than that of zimelidine. Zimelidine, but not imipramine at the corresponding dose, changed the amplitude-intensity slope of the N_{140} component in VEP towards a more pronounced reduction. This effect seems to be due to changes produced in the serotoninergic pathways. The amplitudes or latencies of P_{100}, N_{140} or P_{200} at a stimulus intensity of 0.1 J were not influenced by either imipramine or zimelidine.

References

Coppen, A.; Rama Rao, V.A.; Swade, C.; Wood, K.: Inhibition of 5-hydroxytryptamine reuptake by amitryptiline and zimelidine and its relationship to their therapeutic action. Psychopharmacology *63:* 125–129 (1979).

Gottfries, C.G.; Knorring, L. von; Perris, C.: Neurophysiological measures related to levels of 5-HIAA, HVA and tryptophan in CSF of psychiatric patients. Neuropsychobiology *2:* 1–8 (1976).

Knorring, L. von: Changes in saliva secretion and accommodation width during short-term administration of imipramine and zimelidine in healthy volunteers. Int. Psychopharmacol. *16:* 69–78 (1981).

Knorring, L. von; Johansson, F.; Almay, B.: Augmenting/reducing response in visual evoked potentials in patients with chronic pain syndromes. Adv. biol. Psychiat. *4:* 55–62 (1980).

Knorring, L. von; Mörnstad, H.; Qualitative changes in saliva composition during short-term administration of imipramine and zimelidine in healthy volunteers. Scand. J. dent. Res. *89:* 313–320 (1981).

Knorring, L. von; Perris, C.: Biochemistry of the augmenting-reducing response in visual evoked potentials. Neuropsychobiology *7:* 1–8 (1981).

Redmond, D.E.; Borge, G.F.; Buchsbaum, M.; Maas, J.W.: Evoked potential studies in brain cathecholamine alterations in monkeys. J. psychiat. Res. *12:* 96–116 (1975).

Siwers, B.; Ringberger, V.-A.; Tuck, J.R.; Sjöquist, F.: Initial clinical trial based on biochemical methodology of zimelidine (a serotonin uptake inhibitor) in depressed patients. Clin. Pharmacol. Ther. *21:* 194–200 (1977).

L. von Knorring, MD, Department of Psychiatry, Umeå University, S-90185 Umeå (Sweden)

Subject Index